EveryBody Is A Body

EveryBody **Is A Body**

By Karen A. Studd
& Laura L. Cox

This edition published by
Dog Ear Publishing
4010 W. 86th Street, Ste H
Indianapolis, IN 46268

www.dogearpublishing.net

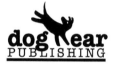

ISBN: 978-145751-850-8
This book is printed on acid-free paper.

Printed in the United States of America

EveryBody **Is A Body**

By Karen A. Studd & Laura L. Cox

Table of Contents

Table of Contents

Table of Contents

Acknowledgements

The authors would like to thank the community of Laban Movement Analysts with whom we are honored to share our passion for this work. We also thank our students who continue to surprise and inspire us. We wish to acknowledge and extend thanks to Rena Milgrom for supporting the publication of this book in the Czech Republic.

A very special thanks goes to Sandra Hooghwinkel for integrating her LMA knowledge and computer expertise in creating the visual design and for finding and creating images for this book. The authors are indebted to Sandra for her integral assistance with this project.

We are grateful to the Laban/Bartenieff Institute of Movement Studies for promoting and supporting the training of Movement Analysts for over thirty years. Thanks to Karen Bradley, for her tireless promotion of LMA and its value in the world. We also want to thank Rachelle Tsachor, Robin Collen and Susan Scarth, CMAs who have used early versions of this book in their programs. For expertise in editing, we thank Douglas Cox.

*EveryBody **Is A Body***

Introduction

This is a book about human movement. *EveryBody **Is A Body*** is a book intended for everyone, whether you are an athlete, a person who tries to avoid moving, or someone who generally gives their movement little thought. Movement is a fundamental fact of our existence, so much so that we lose awareness of its pervasive nature.

This book is not a "how to" book. We are not advocating a specific movement technique or practice. Rather, it is about re-discovering that you are (whether you believe it or not), in fact, a mover. We are always feeling, sensing, creating, connecting and transforming through movement. This book is free of exercise regimens, health recipes or rules for movement. It is about bringing to your conscious attention that which is largely unconscious. It is about recognizing and experiencing yourself through movement.

We are used to thinking of movement only in particular domains, such as sports, fitness and child development. Books on movement reflect our thinking in this way. There are countless books dedicated to particular sports. There are books on the science of movement: kinesiology, motor development and anatomy/physiology. There are books on the art of movement: theater and dance. There are books on specialized movement practices such as yoga, Pilates and martial art forms. There are even books on "body language", recognizing the power and potential of nonverbal communication.

There are relatively few books, however, that address the ubiquitous nature of movement that connects us all – from Olympic athletes to couch potatoes, from operatic singers to singers in the shower, from the physical laborers of Main Street to the CEOs of Wall Street. For everybody, movement is the basis of functional and expressive life.

Having been engaged in the process of writing this book for several years, we now have a profound appreciation for the reasons why so few books on the big picture of human movement exist. We discovered that trying to verbalize something that is non-verbal is hugely challenging. More importantly, trying to address the omnipresent nature of movement is like asking a fish to describe the water in which he is swimming! When we started this process, we also fell into a niche of writing about a movement specialization. As teachers in a specialized program for analyzing human movement, we began by writing what we felt was a much-needed textbook. Our initial efforts were to create an overall text of the theory and practice of Laban Movement Analysis and Bartenieff Fundamentals™ (LMA/BF).

In our efforts to write that text, over and over again, we found ourselves asking, why is the LMA/BF system for the study of movement known to so few? In attempting to answer that question, we bumped up against another – why is it so difficult to describe the field of movement study to those who have never heard of it? As we considered these questions, we began to realize that the answer could be found in the fact that **movement is the foundation of life.**

Introduction

Because movement is so basic, pervasive and ephemeral, we lose conscious awareness of it. Moreover, contemporary culture reinforces this loss of movement awareness. As technology expands, so too does disembodiment. Advanced technology is designed to remove us from body experience as we rely upon machines to do more and more physical work, and as we increasingly connect in the virtual environments of the Internet and wireless technology. While the upside of this is obvious, there is an alarming downside. As areas of human endeavor become increasingly specialized, human movement becomes more diminished and compartmentalized. The result of this is a disconnection from one's body, and by extension, disconnection from one's physical existence. This in turn leads to discomfort, a sense of not feeling comfortable in one's own skin, and can progress to actual chronic pain syndromes and "dis-ease".

We hope this book brings awareness of the greater Body of Knowledge that is human movement and provides individuals with increased awareness of the power and potential of their own movement. We want all our fellow movers to experience the pleasure and ease of the moving body. This is a book for every body. We all move. All of the time. This has meaning. It is vitally important not to lose touch with our moving selves.

Books on specific movement applications tell just a piece of the story. Texts on kinesiology and fitness focus on the functional aspects of movement. Books on movement for actors and body language focus on expressive aspects. In recent years, many books have appeared that address aspects of somatic practices. Somatic practice is based on the philosophy that Body/Mind/Spirit are interconnected, and encourages the process of self-exploration through body awareness. However, books on somatics are generally written for a population that already has some investment and experience in the field. The readers these books tend to attract include movement therapists, movement educators, "hands on" healers or students who are already steeped in knowledge of movement. However, such books can be off-putting for much of the general population, who may find the material out of their comfort zone. We hope to make consciousness of movement accessible to everyone while avoiding the pitfall of writing too simplistically.

Words alone are inadequate to express fully the experience that is movement. Poets and philosophers have bravely tried to grapple with this – but very few others! While it is difficult to describe movement through language, paradoxically our language reveals the pervasiveness of movement. The primary way in which language does this is through metaphor based on the experience of the body. To illustrate just how commonplace body metaphors are, throughout the text we have highlighted them in red (as we did above with the metaphor Body of Knowledge.) In addition to connecting language and movement, and because this is a book about movement, throughout the book we encourage the reader to experience simple movements that illustrate the concepts we discuss. These experiences are highlighted in blue and are labeled "Try This". Don't worry! These "Try This" directions are easily accomplished, even while reading the book.

As professionals in the field of movement, the authors not only teach in the Laban/Bartenieff training programs, we work with students and clients in a variety of contexts to enhance and optimize their individual movement potential. Our work ranges from alleviating stress and chronic pain, to facilitating public speaking, to improving the technique of dancers and athletes. In all these contexts, we seek to assist the individual in becoming aware of habitual movement patterns and preferences. We draw from our backgrounds as dancers, educators, movement analysts and somatics practitioners. We believe the moving self reflects the Whole self. Although humans share the same design and basic anatomy, each body is also individually unique. EveryBody expresses who they are functionally, intellectually and emotionally through movement. Our moving selves reflect the culture in which we were raised, our values, our upbringing, and the tools we choose to navigate through the world. Even people with physical limitations move. A person with severe arthritis still uses movement both functionally and expressively. Choosing when, how, and even *if* to move reveals something about the nature of that individual.

The authors have named their approach to movement re-education **WholeMovement.** This approach takes into account the nature of common anatomical design while honoring the uniqueness of every individual. The **WholeMovement** approach, which is based primarily on Laban Movement Analysis and Bartenieff Fundamentals™, supports the experience of the Wholeness of self through movement. Throughout this book we emphasize the importance of integration and Wholeness by capitalizing the word Whole wherever it appears.

The benefits of becoming conscious of the Wholeness of your moving self can be transformative. You can gain greater insight about who you are from how you move. Our movement results from our genetic predispositions, our cultural heritage, individual family dynamics, daily activities, the choices we make and much more. All of these factors contribute to one's unique movement signature. Knowing something about who you are as a mover leads to greater knowledge about who you are as a person.

Over the course of one's lifetime, movement awareness contributes to health and well-being, helping to avoid stress and situations that may lead to chronic pain and disease. Self-awareness also supports our interactions with others. Personal insights from awareness of your movement patterns allow you to control and modify your behaviors and empathize with the patterns of others. Movement is not just a body activity. It is the expression of our Whole selves in connection with the world.

* Laban Movement Analysis and Bartenieff Fundamentals™ (LMA/BF) is a comprehensive system for the observation and analysis of movement. This system is structured on the work of the early 20th century artist and visionary Rudolf Laban. The system has been further developed by his followers, including: Irmgard Bartenieff, Warren Lamb, Judith Kestenberg, Martha Davis, Peggy Hackney and many others. The system utilizes specific terminology, which appears in capital letters when referenced in the text of this book. For further information on LMA/BF, contact the Laban/Bartenieff Institute of Movement Studies (LIMS) @limsonline.org

Chapter 1

What is Movement?

Becoming Conscious of Your Moving Self

Why Become Conscious of Your Moving Self?

How Do We Define Movement?

The Basic Patterns

The Body as Basis of Duality

The Flow of Change

The *What,* the *Where* and the *How* of Movement

What is Basic?

Chapter 1

What Is Movement?

"All things change, nothing is extinguished. There is nothing in the whole world which is permanent. Everything flows onward; all things are brought into being with a changing nature; the ages themselves glide by in constant movement."
Ovid

Becoming Conscious of Your Moving Self

Right now what are you doing? Are your eyes moving to track the words on this page? What position are you in? Are you still or are you shifting weight, brushing hair out of your eyes, tapping your foot? If you perceive yourself to be still, change to a new position. What did you choose to do? How is it different (or is it)? Can you sense the fourth toe of your right foot? Did you have to move to find it?

One of the things we do throughout the day is continually readjust our body's position. We cross and uncross our legs as we sit. While standing in line we shift weight from one foot to the other. We moisten our lips, rub our hands together; the list of examples is endless. Whether these adjustments are obvious or subtle, they are part of the continuous conversation of the body with itself. This subtle, and sometimes not so subtle, adjustment of our positions keeps us connected to ourselves and helps us to self-assess. We also check in with ourselves through our actions of self-touch as we rub our hands together, massage a sore spot or run our fingers through our hair. This self-monitoring is a vital part of self-maintenance and is crucial to our well-being. However, we frequently do not receive or attend to the signals we are sending ourselves.

The negative consequences of sitting at a computer for hours on end are well known and we are instructed by health advocates to take a break, take a walk, find a good chair or a better keyboard. These are good suggestions, but are not always possible and often seem prescriptive (yet another task to accomplish). All too often, these suggestions are too little too late, because neck pain and general discomfort probably have already set in. So, while you are working, choose to become consciously aware of your body by taking advantage of your built in capacity to monitor and make adjustments. Don't wait until you feel discomfort. Perhaps you could regularly shake out your hands, turn your head away from the computer screen, shrug your shoulders, sigh (really sigh – audibly), close your eyes, yawn (the possibilities for relief are endless and specific to you and your personal needs). One person's choice might be to allow himself to passively become limp and slack. Another person might choose to actively hum and bounce. A third person might decide to stand up and stretch, then shake-out before he sits back down. Do something that feels good, not just something that you "should" do.

The key is to tap into the sensation of the body, to check in with yourself and what you are doing. While operating in a thinking mode, we do not have to cut off sensation, although we frequently do. And indeed, our sensing and thinking modes support each other and promote balance between the exertions and recuperations built into life. When you invite friends to dinner and stimulating conversation, you are inviting them to feed both their thinking and sensing selves.

What are you aware of when you first wake up in the morning? Are you already in your head thinking about your "to do" list? Or are you in your body, connected to sensations indicating revitalized energy or continued fatigue? While there are different types of consciousness, the thinking mode predominates. We also tend to compartmentalize our thoughts, sensations and emotions as if they were discreet processes. Becoming conscious of yourself as a mover involves fully experiencing your sensing self. The sensing self, the thinking self, and the feeling self are parts of the Whole self. Connecting all these parts of ourselves is how we find the Wholeness of ourselves.

Why Become Conscious of your Moving Self?

Conscious awareness of your movement is vital to experiencing the Wholeness of your life. However, if this is the case, then why don't we do this? In part, the simple answer is because we couldn't function if we had to be conscious of our movement constantly. If we had to be aware of every step in a simple process such as getting dressed in the morning, it would take all our time and energy! For instance, describing every action required to put on a pair of socks might go something like this:

> *Assuming you have already chosen the socks you will wear, begin by extending your dominant hand toward a sock. Modify your hand/eye tracking to make sure your hand actually connects with the sock. Open the fingers of your hand then continue by shaping your hand around the sock. Close your fingers to grasp the sock. Retract your arm toward the body. Now change your focus and direct it towards the foot. Bend the trunk to incline the upper body toward the foot. With both hands, grasp the opening of the sock while flexing at the ankle to lift the toes off the floor. Place the opening of the sock over the toes and gently pull the sock toward the back of the foot. Now lift the heel off the floor, continue to pull the sock up over the heel and ankle. Put the foot back on the floor and release the hands. Bring the torso back to an upright position. Repeat the process with the other sock on the other foot. Note: you may have a personal sock ritual that differs from this. We chose a very simplified description, and left out several steps related to starting position, postural changes, gesture, focus, modulation of muscular tensions, etc. Whew!*

Enough already. There is good reason for much of our movement to become habitual patterns that we no longer need to think about. It frees us to attend to other things (like building a better mousetrap or presenting a case to the Supreme Court). There is a dark side, however. Loss of awareness of ourselves as movers can lead to a variety of "bad habits" affecting our health and well being. In order to recognize habits, whether "good" or "bad", one first has to become conscious of them. Awareness gives you the option to modify habits, if needed.

Much of our movement begins with motivation – whether conscious or not. All living creatures move from a basic motivation to survive. From the imperative to survive to the simple pleasure of tapping the fingers in time to music, all movement begins as response to stimulus. For example, a baby lying on his belly hears a sound that motivates him to turn his head, which may then result in his rolling over onto his back. If this response is a positive outcome for the infant (he sees his mother making the sound) he will be apt to repeat that movement. Repetition does for the nervous system what water does to rock over time. Pathways of response become carved out, making repetition more and more likely. This eventually leads to patterned movement. What was once intentional eventually becomes a habit that no longer requires conscious awareness. Think about a child learning to tie his shoes. Much like our sock example, initially the child must give his full conscious attention to each step of this movement sequence, but over time it can be done in a flash with little or no conscious thought process.

The downside of losing conscious awareness of most movement is that we are also unaware of movement patterns that don't serve us well. We may have developed patterns that contribute to fatigue and chronic pain, and even interfere with our ability to relate to others. Why, you might wonder, would we have an inefficient pattern? There are several possibilities. For example, perhaps you learned as a child that you could concentrate better when listening to directions by closing your eyes to cut off extraneous visual cues. Now as an adult, you have a habit of closing your eyes at times when someone is speaking to you. This habit may lead to someone feeling slighted that you are not paying adequate attention to her, or even that you are being rude.

In another example, a simple postural habit arises in a woman who carries a shoulder bag always on the same shoulder. To keep the bag from slipping off, she hikes the shoulder up toward her ear. The muscles adapt to this unbalanced position and may over time lead to chronic neck, shoulder and back pain.

If the movers in both examples above can become conscious of their movement patterns, they may make a conscious choice to do something else. The woman with the shoulder bag could choose to alternate shoulders for carrying, or change the shoulder bag to a backpack. In both cases, the mover makes a conscious choice to change a pattern. By reawakening awareness of our movement, we may be free again to choose the movement that best supports us.

In order to become aware of movement, we need to start by understanding what movement is. But what, exactly, is movement?

How do we Define Movement?

To fully grasp how fundamental movement is, look it up in the dictionary. You will see that the dictionary uses *movement* to define movement! According to Webster's New World International Dictionary, **movement** is:

1. Moving or a manner of *moving*
2. An *evacuation* of the bowels
3. A *change* in the location of troops

4. Organized *action* by people working toward a goal
5. The *moving* parts of a mechanism as of a clock

and the definition of the verb, to **move,** is no more enlightening:

1. To *change* the place or position
2. To *change* one's residence
3. To be *active*
4. To *make* progress
5. To *take action*
6. To set or be set in *motion*
7. To *arouse*

The common denominator in all of the above definitions is "change", and change is only possible through the process of movement. When something moves, a change occurs. When something has changed, it has moved.

Now, if everything is moving all of the time, this sounds like complete chaos. How do we deal with all of this ongoing movement all around us? In making sense of our environment, humans create order from the patterns of change that they perceive and experience. We feel hot and we feel cold, we move right and we move left. We understand these conditions relative to one another, from the process of change from hot to cold or from side to side. As we cope with and master the world around us, we do so by discerning the patterns of change in the constant movement of life, from the smallest patterns to the largest. Human beings make sense of the world through this ordering of the patterns of change. We categorize these patterns in such things as growth, reproduction, and evolution. From our experience of the movement of our bodies, we organize and expand our perceptions into our knowing and understanding the world around us.

Starting from subatomic particles that are defined by their patterns of movement, to the molecular structure of matter, to the organization of organic and inorganic matter, to the geological organization of the planet from its core to atmosphere, from the cellular structure of organisms, to living systems of multi-cellular organisms, to the organization of organisms into groups, to human evolution, to the timeline of human history with its socio-technological development, to the movement of the planet to the movement of the solar system to the movement of the cosmos, all is defined through changes that we organize and identify as patterns.

According to Albert Einstein, "Nothing changes until something moves". Therefore we propose the following definition of movement: **Patterns of Change**.

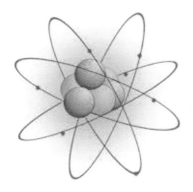

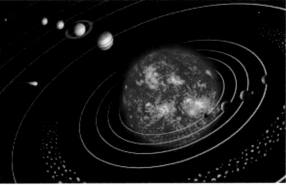

Atomic particles   Planets orbiting

The Basic Patterns

How do we identify patterns? Patterns are repetitive units that make sense. There are patterns of nature that can be recognized from the smallest units such as the arrangement of the chemical elements in the Periodic Table; to larger units such as the grouping of life into categories from Kingdom through Species. We are able to recognize patterns through the process of repetition.

When we perceive the sequence of a pattern, we can describe this pattern as a phrase. Sequence creates a progression from beginning to end. Phrases are parts of a bigger Whole, but are complete within themselves. Phrases, whether in music, speech or movement, connect to other phrases to form a larger meaning and are a basic pattern of organization. We see phrases in both larger and smaller patterns. We can see the phrase of a life as beginning with birth and ending with death. Within the large phrase of an individual life, we identify smaller sub-phrases, from childhood to old age.

In a phrase, beginning and end have a relationship in the progression of time. This relationship is fundamental to the basic pattern of development. All development, whether technological or biological, is movement; patterns of change through a progression of time.

Another basic pattern we identify is duality. This pattern starts from the perceptual process of differentiating something from what it is not. The organizing pattern of duality furthers the foundation for making sense of our world and is a vital strategy of our development and our survival. We identify **self** from **other**, decide on the necessary course of action in **fight** or **flight** and determine what is **edible** from what is **inedible**. We organize the passage of time into now and then, day and night, past and future. We organize our self in relationship to our environment - through here and there, toward and away, in and out. We continually organize our perceptions through dualities of hot and cold, strong and weak, loud and quiet, smooth and rough, sweet and sour, and on and on.

To summarize, the basic patterns we have identified include phrasing, developmental progression, and duality.

The Body as Basis of Duality

Starting with our body at its simplest level of duality, even the cell functions by differentiating what is contained within the cell wall from what is not. In human development, one of the fundamental dualities is the distinction between Self and Other.

Through our perceptions and the experience of our bodies, we create this idea of duality, designating polar opposites existing on a continuum. While we do identify opposites, opposites are in fact two aspects of a greater Whole. Hot and cold are two ends of a temperature continuum. Up and down are two ends of a spatial continuum. Inside and outside are relative to each other. The concept of duality is a paradox. Opposites do not cancel each other out, but rather, they support each other and exist simultaneously. We can only understand "up" because there is a "down". As the sculptor Henry Moore said, "To know one thing, you must know the opposite". Human beings are pattern makers. We deconstruct the ongoing experience of life to create patterns that allow us to navigate and interact. In seeing the patterns, it is important not to lose awareness of how they form the Whole.

Through our moving bodies we identify many patterns of duality. We experience the pull of gravity as down versus up, we experience breathing in and breathing out, we experience ourselves as awake or asleep, we have a right side and a left side, we have a front and a back. We assign labels of duality relative to these experiences of the body. We identify the opposites of right and left based on our bilateral symmetry. We differentiate front from back relative to the placement of our eyes and the organization of our joints for locomotion. We differentiate hot and cold based on body sensation. Temperature is only hot when it is considered relative to something colder. Hot and cold are not actual entities, they are conditions we initially designate based on sensation. Through the filter of our perceptions, we assign dualities as a way to make sense of our experience.

The Flow of Change

We are born into the ongoingness of life. This ongoingness can be recognized as the flow of life. The word flow in one of its many definitions is "to move with a continual change of place among the constituent particles or parts". So, within the larger flow of a river, the individual water molecules are moving together. The moving of these parts creates a Whole, through which we perceive flow. The movement of individual vehicles on the highway results in the flow of traffic. A field of wheat appears to flow in the wind. Everything flows!

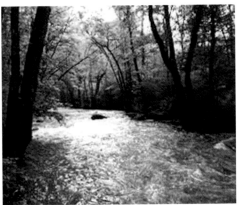
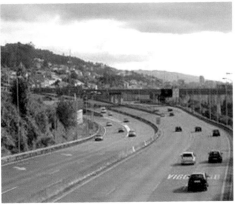

Flowing river   *Vehicular flow of traffic*

Everything moves, so everything is participating in the universal process of flow. We experience flow because we are living bodies changing through the abundance of physiological processes occurring in an uninterrupted streaming until the day of death. Thoughts flow as neurons fire in the cerebral cortex; blood flows in a pulsating rhythm of energy exchange; the flow of digestion carries nutrients into the body and expels waste. All these inner (micro) flows contribute to the larger (macro) flow of the body as a Whole flowing through space. And this gives way to larger flows of groups of bodies in societies and civilizations through time. (The progression of time itself is perceived as flow). This understanding of flow can be aligned with the concept of Chi – the circulating life force that underlies Chinese philosophy and medicine.

Flow immediately brings to mind images of water. These images arise directly from our primordial evolution from water to land, as well as from our embryonic existence in the fluid-filled womb. We know that life on earth arose from the sea and our individual entrance to the world is heralded by the "breaking of the waters" when we are born. It may be that the experience of flow is the fundamental commonality among all living organisms. From this perspective, flow can be seen as the stream from which empathy arises. We can connect to another's experience and take it on as if it were our own. This ability to become one with another being is rooted in the biochemistry of emotion which we define as feeling. Recent developments in the study of the phenomena of mirror neurons appear to support that our bodies are patterned to connect with others.

Emotional feelings arise from changes in bodily sensation, which reflect changes in bodily flow: quickening heartbeat, sweaty palms, hair raising, dry mouth. We actually describe emotions with respect to the bodily events with which they are associated. An adventure is spine tingling. A parting is heart wrenching. A side splitting joke tickles our fancy. A beautiful sunset takes our breath away. We shake in our boots, and feel butterflies in our stomach. An insult leaves a bad taste in our mouth. Changes in bodily sensations are what lead to "feelings" that we identify as emotions.

Our individual flow is born of, and depends upon, the larger flow of life. The process of learning and developing can be boiled down to the process of gaining increased control over our flow. Babies are little containers of potential in motion. Motor development progresses from the organization of our core to our limbs, from gross muscle movement to the more finely tuned and complex patterns, which will eventually let us type at the computer and dance the tango. Even though one can discuss motor development as if it were a separate component of personal development, it actually is part of an integrated Whole. As we develop control of our limbs, we are also developing the ability to control our emotions, master our intellect, and negotiate relationships with others.

Flow can be understood as the energetic continuum from completely unrestrained chaos to rigidity. As we develop we are learning to manipulate flow, to negotiate the balance of flow among differing life contexts as needed. The ability to modify our flow enables us to accomplish different goals. Flow serves us both functionally as well as expressively. For example, inserting a contact lens requires the mover to control flow to place the lens on the delicate and small surface of the eye. In a larger context, our use of flow also serves us expressively. When you advise someone to "just let it go", you are advising them to release the constraint of the flow of emotions such as frustration. While sometimes it is valuable to show restraint in our actions (control of flow), at other times it might be beneficial to take a leap of faith (release of flow).

Flow as energetic life force connects our inner world flow to the outer world flow. We are involved in a constant give and take between our energy flowing outward and the energy of the world streaming into and around us. This is true even with the fundamental process of breathing: we inhale the outer world and exhale our inner world.

The control of flow is necessary for communicating and relating. Binding flow creates boundaries that can be more or less appropriate according to the nature of the relationship. Freeing flow permeates boundaries, allowing for greater intimacy in relationships. An appropriate control of flow helps to clarify relationships among individuals in all contexts.

As we learn to control flow we are essentially patterning our flow. Patterns of flow are uniquely individual and underlie our sense of self. As we stated earlier, the body flowing within itself is constantly adapting, shifting and self assessing. This ongoing conversation of self-flow can be seen as part of the distinctive movement signature of every individual. Countless little self-referencing movements (like how someone runs her fingers through her hair) are part of how we recognize each other. Self-flow (termed Shape Flow in LMA) is part of the blueprint for impersonators, enabling them to capture the essence of someone.

From this flow of the self, to the flow that bridges self to other, to the flow of mutual interaction, life can be seen as a progression from the undefined wriggling of infancy, to the highly refined articulation of a surgeon's hands. Because the ongoing flow of movement permeates and surrounds us like water surrounds fish, we lose conscious awareness of it.

The *What* the *Where* and the *How* of Movement: Re-awakening our Movement Awareness

In order to become aware of our movement, we first have to be aware of *what* is moving – our body. The design of our human form, the body, is a given. What we describe as life is the experience of sensation, interpretation, and reaction resulting from the experience of our bodies in the world.

Our human form, starting with its upright posture, aligned with the pull of gravity, our bilateral symmetry and the position of our eyes and ears, determines the nature of our understanding and, in essence, creates our world. If we, for example, walked on four feet instead of two, everything from our architecture to our social rituals would be quite different. As four-legged creatures, we would have created an entirely different world. In this scenario, the meaning and expression of both the power handshake and the Parthenon is gone. Gone too, are the ways in which our metaphors give meaning to our experience. As a quadruped, spatial references such as looking up to someone or rising to the occasion would have different meanings!

The body, or *what* is moving, also determines the *where* of movement. Where we move is built upon our human form, defining what is up, down, right, left, forward or back. The body also determines the *how* of movement, determining the amount and quality of energetic engagement involved in an action. The qualitative components, or dynamics of movement, are an essential aspect of the expressiveness of movement. Expression, whether in tone of voice or in a musical composition, in large part is determined by qualitative change. Speaking loudly or whispering conveys different meanings in the same way fortissimo or pianissimo color the music. A delicate gesture versus a forceful gesture support different intents. Becoming more conscious of *what, where* and *how* we are moving helps to clarify our movement.

Our body is home base and the way in which we know all that we know. In order to become conscious of movement, let's start by exploring the basics of the moving body – the *what, where* and *how* of movement. In order to do this, we don't need to go to the gym, employ personal trainers or buy fancy work-out machines. Just like Dorothy in "The Wizard of Oz" we have always had the power to return home!

What is Basic?

The basics are the "givens" of human existence; we inhabit a world where we breathe in oxygen from the air of the earth's atmosphere and are bound by the pull of gravity and the laws of physics. Anatomically we have evolved into bipedal creatures, who stand and move from an upright posture. Our large complex brains have necessitated a long period of childhood and our opposable thumbs have contributed to our capacity to build and use tools. The environment we inhabit and our biological design are our foundation.

These fundamentals of our existence dictate the essential components of our survival. We need to breathe. We need to eat, to find shelter and to interact with other people. And in fulfilling any of our survival needs - we move. The movement of our bodies is essential to survival. The movement of our bodies is basic to life.

Breathing is a primary movement pattern of every individual. Upon birth, our first breath marks our entry into the world as a unique person. This largely unconscious action supports every aspect of our life. Our cells receive oxygen from breath. The ability to vocalize (whether giving directions or singing an aria) depends on breath. Breath is at the heart of our emotional life. We express ourselves with sighs of ecstasy and groans of despair. Many spiritual practices address the power of breath. Take a moment to become aware of the fact that you are breathing right now. Reflect on the fact that we breathe all day long, 24/7, for the duration of life. We take this basic for granted, unless there is a problem such as asthma or allergies.

Survival, both for early man and his modern descendants, requires the movement of our bodies. We move to transport ourselves from one location to another. We move to hunt and gather (whether in the fields or the local market). We move in order to make and use tools. Even after meeting our survival needs, our higher needs too, require movement to be fulfilled. A painter, a surgeon, an architect, a musician all use body movement to achieve their goals. What is the movement specific to the work that you do? Even those with desk jobs must move their body to get the job done.

Man is, by his nature, a social being. It is through the palette of our movement that we interact with others and express our individuality. Although we move as individuals, we also move together when we make love, raise children and build bridges and institutions. We work and play in community. Where do you move in community with others? At church? At the bowling alley? At a sporting event or other performance?

It is through the movement of breath, through our everyday functional movement, and the movement of interaction with others, that we define ourselves. Although it seems obvious that we breathe, that we move, that we interact: we lose conscious awareness of the patterns of movement that define our lives. Try this: now that you have finished reading this chapter, become aware of what your sensations are and how you are feeling. What movement would feel good to do right now? Would you like to reposition yourself? Stand up and shake out? Change your eye focus? Stretch? Why not do it?

Taking a moment to breathe, and to bring to conscious awareness what you are doing (moving) gives EveryBody the opportunity to focus, to recuperate, to prepare, and to communicate more effectively. When we become more self aware we optimize our ability to live our lives to the fullest extent.

Chapter 2

Language & Movement:
Two Parts of the Whole

The Verbal/Nonverbal Split

Right Brain/Left Brain – Two Sides of the Whole

Meaning and Metaphor

The Body/Mind Duality Fallacy

Understanding Movement through Themes of Duality

Function/Expression

Stability/Mobility

Exertion/Recuperation

Inner/Outer

Dualities within Wholeness

Chapter 2

Language & Movement:
Two Parts Of The Whole

"Movement is one of man's languages and as such it must be consciously mastered."
Rudolf Laban

Our body is both the container and contents of all our experience that transpires from our birth until our death. This reality is shared by all humans. Our bodies are humanity's common denominator. They are our common bond. The body expresses our individual uniqueness as well as the primal universal aspect of what it means to be human. The body is the starting point of the shared experience of being human, all of us inhabiting a form shaped by a common ancestry.

We live *through* our bodies, we live *with* our bodies. Our bodies provide the means to take in (perceive), connect and interact with the world. Knowing is based in experience and experience is embodied. Let's emphasize this – **experience is embodied.** All experience is that of the living body, and this is the experience of movement.

Movement is what defines reality as we know it and construct it – whether it be the movement of the cosmos or the movement of subatomic particles, everything is defined and categorized by its movement. We are driven to move. Motivation provides intent and intent is taken into action. This is true whether you are young or old, male or female, from the East or from the West, able-bodied and athletic or feeble and infirm.

We humans, because of our survival needs, for subsistence and protection, are instinctively social creatures. Thus a large part of the history of our evolution includes the development of our capacity to communicate with others: both to express ourselves and to understand the expression of others. The necessity to coexist with others has contributed to, and to large extent, determines our verbal and non-verbal behaviors. How and why our bodies convey and interpret information is the foundation of human expression and communication.

From our experience of our bodies in relationship to the environment and other people, we create meaning. Meaning-making occurs through our ability to make connections among these experiences. The reason we assign meaning is to communicate shared experience. This process connects to the development of language. In other words, language evolves from our movement experience. It is not separate from movement, but rather an extension of movement.

The Verbal/Nonverbal Split

Language grows out of movement. Just as an apple is related to the tree that produced it, language is a part of the experience of movement. However, the verbal and non-verbal domains have been separated and compartmentalized. Isolating the parts of something is a methodology leading to understanding. We pull things apart in order to figure them out. This is how bodies of knowledge have been built, delineated and added to throughout history. It is why science is now separate from philosophy and art. It is why you may go to a medical specialist rather than a general practitioner – or why you call a plumber rather than simply a handy man.

Through the analytical process, patterns are recognized and categorized. This discernment starts from a comparative process of sorting what something "is" from what it is "not". This process of comparison is grounded in our primary duality: Self/Not Self. This necessary Self/Other separation starts us down the road of the human condition. It leads to knowledge and understanding, as well as to isolation. A short distance down this road, language is defined as one thing and movement, another. The notion of verbal and nonverbal as separate entities comes into being.

Our conscious perception generally places our verbal side prominently in the foreground. The nonverbal side is left almost completely unattended in the background of our perception. This separation of Verbal Self from Nonverbal Self is aligned with the experience of a Mind/Body split. Our thinking self is perceived as being separate from the sensorial experience of the body. Of course, it is not. Verbal and Nonverbal are two parts of a Whole.

Right Brain/Left Brain – Two Sides of the Whole

A characteristic in our human design emphasizing both duality and Wholeness is the hemispheric lateralization of our brains. Bi-lobed brains are found in all vertebrates. However in humans, the two brain hemispheres are functionally different from each other. This duality is unlike having two kidneys, where both are functionally the same. The functional differentiation of our brain came about through the process of our evolution and is linked to our language development, capacity for abstract thinking, and much of what makes us extremely versatile and adaptable beings.

In the majority of the population (those who are right handed), the left brain is the center of analytical, linear thinking. It is the location of language skills and the ego of self and of exerting the will of self. The left brain is the center of "doing" in extending the self through creating and manipulating tools.

The right brain, older developmentally than the left side, is the home of facial recognition and it is associated with nonverbal aspects of communication and perception. It is the locus of intuition and associated with our gut response. It is emotional rather than analytical and, rather than "doing" it is concerned with "being". The right brain is the realm of imagery, mystery and faith, not logic and numbers.

16

The complex nature of our brains is due in part to the differentiation of the two hemispheres. This differentiation assigns independent functions to each side, allowing the two sides to work separately. In addition, each side is also capable of taking on some functions of the opposite side when needed. For example, in cases where injury to one side of the brain has occurred, the other side has the capacity to adapt, taking on some of the lost function to maintain Wholeness. The capacity of the two hemispheres of our brain to act independently, to be malleable, and to connect and interact contributes to the vast capacity of the human mind and our seemingly endless potential.

A cornerstone of the synergistic connection between the right and left sides of the brain is the phenomenon of metaphor. Metaphor is a form of speech, but one that draws its power from imagery arising from physical experience. Metaphor gives words the power to transcend the linear logical nature of the language construct. The use of metaphor demonstrates the integration of the two sides of our brain and is a great definer of the human experience.

Meaning and Metaphor

The power of language is built from the power of words. Words are tools that we use to express ourselves and communicate, also to think and analyze. When you name something, you take control of it. Naming bestows power. The power of naming can be seen archetypically throughout the course of history, from Adam naming the animals in the Garden of Eden to Harry Potter giving voice to the name of the evil Voldemort.

A significant aspect of our languaging incorporates metaphor. And a dominant characteristic of metaphor is that it arises from our bodily experience. Metaphors are perhaps the most fundamental way in which we organize the *patterns* of our experience. Metaphors are so omnipresent that we are not even aware of how often we use references to body experience in daily communication. In fact, while writing this book the authors have enjoyed continuously being reminded of the body/movement metaphors so frequently used in everyday language.

Take a moment to think about what is being described when someone says they feel down. The posture of someone who feels down is generally drooping, the body's weight collapsing into gravity. Perhaps their eyes are down cast, and their shoulders are slumped. What about the person who is feeling up? Have their spirits been lifted? Do they feel on top of the world? In all likelihood, their posture is buoyant and more vertically upright.

Some ways in which metaphor grows out of body experience include:

- Our organization of space (for instance, we talk about looking up to someone or looking down on someone)

- Our organization of body parts (we describe something as heart breaking or someone as spineless)

- Our organization of perception (characterizing something as touching or in poor taste)

- Our metaphors of simple movement actions (describing someone as pushy, or being urged to stand up to your boss, or giving someone the brush off)

The list of metaphors based in the experience of the body is endless. Try this: read any article in a newspaper or magazine and see how many times there is a metaphoric reference to the experience of our human form. If you don't see any on the first try, read it again. Becoming conscious takes practice!

The power of language is generally well understood. The power of movement generally is not. Movement, when acknowledged, is given an isolated peripheral role. Movement study, by and large, is limited to areas such as Physical Education. In college theater departments, specialized classes in Movement for Actors are offered. This nomenclature says it all, implying that movement as an aspect of education is somehow separate from other aspects of education. Movement as an overarching idea is virtually unknown and it continues to be addressed peripherally through specialized skills in areas such as sports, dance, gymnastics, stage combat, martial arts, etc. These specializations are generally considered as supplemental or elective, and are the first to be cut when budgets are strained.

On one hand it is said that, "the pen is mightier than the sword". On the other hand, it is also said that, "actions speak louder than words". Movement and language are not separate entities. They are two parts of an integrated Whole. To use a metaphor, movement is at the heart of our language. From the experience of our bodies we create ever more complex levels of abstraction, which refer back to concrete fundamental body experience. Unfortunately, as our language skills develop, the body knowledge which led to these skills is submerged. In other words, we lose conscious awareness of movement when language comes to the forefront of consciousness. Part of this loss of awareness is losing sight of the fact that speaking is moving! The production of spoken language requires the highly articulated physical actions of the mouth, tongue, and muscles of the face. Movement is fundamental in speech therapy and in public speaking. It is through the re-integration of the verbal and nonverbal parts of ourselves that we may best achieve cohesive Wholeness.

The Mind/Body Duality Fallacy

The Verbal/Nonverbal duality designation is an aspect of the Mind/Body schism. As with all dualities, the seemingly opposite sides are actually two parts of a greater Whole. We generally associate language with the thinking, conscious part of ourselves. In contrast, the nonverbal part of ourselves is associated with the body. While these associations are valid, they limit the Wholeness of our knowing. Remember that language develops from the movement of the body. We are only able to think because we have a body to think through. The notion of the body and mind as separate entities is a hallmark of Western thought. Even today, when developments in neuroscience provide evidence of the Wholeness of body and mind, those seeking to cling to the distinction of body and mind do this by separating the anatomy of the brain from the mind.

In Eastern philosophy and medicine, the body and mind are not artificially separated. The classic example of this is the symbol of Yin/Yang. The two parts are contained within one circle. The two parts form a Whole. While there has been growing interest in holistic wellness, along with a rise of interest in Eastern practices such as yoga, acupuncture and Tai Chi, Western thought still predominates in how we live our lives. Attending a yoga class and becoming aware of your breathing is a good start, but it doesn't undo centuries of a Cartesian world-view. As you may recall, Rene Descartes was the 17th Century philosopher who is known for the saying, "I think, therefore, I am". *The truth is, we think because we are.*

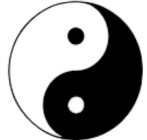

Understanding Movement through Themes of Duality

The nature of Wholeness rests in the balance and integration of dualities. Although examples of patterns of duality in life can be endlessly listed, Laban Movement Analysis identifies four specific overarching dual movement themes. These include:

- the relationship between Function/Expression
- the rhythms of Exertion/Recuperation
- the interplay between our Inner/Outer worlds
- how we both Mobilize/Stabilize our ever-moving lives

Remember that dualities help us to recognize patterns by separating the Whole into opposing parts. In order to understand movement, the parts must be re-integrated. This process starts with awareness.

Function/Expression

Functional movement (such as thigh flexion) and expressive action (such as literally jumping for joy) are generally viewed as two distinct aspects of physical movement. This is a fallacy that, in part, explains why there is no such thing as a "quick fix" for body related problems. Function is related to the mechanics of movement – it is the part of movement that can be analyzed scientifically, it is the quantifiable, the "what" of movement. Expression is linked to the how and the why of movement.

For example, in order to lose weight, one is advised on a functional level to reduce caloric intake and/or increase energy expenditure. Calories consumed and expended are measurable. There are lots of people who successfully lose weight on diets through this functional approach. However, overwhelming evidence suggests that a majority of these people regain the weight after a period of time. Why? What is missing?

In order for change to be successful, there must be a change in how you perceive yourself and how you choose to express yourself in the world. Unless one is able to make a fundamental shift in the expressive part of oneself, old patterns will reassert themselves. Successful change includes both the purely functional as well as the expressive parts of self. Because our expressive self is not quantifiable, it is harder to acknowledge and therefore, harder to change. For instance, in order to lose weight, perhaps you need to change your self-image from a passive one to an active one. Dieting would not be such a pervasive cultural issue if the "quick fix" of altering the ratio of intake/output were actually the answer.

Success stories of former couch potatoes or recovering addicts share a common theme. These individuals relate that their entire beings changed, not simply a functional aspect of behavior. Their relationships to themselves, to others and to the world, changed. They successfully re-patterned themselves both functionally and expressively.

Stability/Mobility

Newtonian physics tells us that stability and mobility are inversely proportional. In other words, the more stable something is, the less mobile it is. However, consider a stone. It appears to be a stable, immobile structure but actually, on the atomic level it is highly mobile. Everything is both stable and mobile in varying degrees, and relative to point of view. In terms of human movement, stability and mobility are directly proportional. To be stable, there must be mobility as underlying support. To be mobile, there must be a stable foundation.

We tend to operate under the assumption that we either "hold on" or "let go". But paradoxically, to do one, you must on some level do the other as well. Everyone has had the experience of trying to balance, whether it be standing on one leg or riding a bicycle. If you try to hold on by clenching your muscles, holding your breath and locking into a position in an effort to stabilize, you will fall over! Successful balance is achieved by going with the ever-changing flux of our inherently mobile selves.

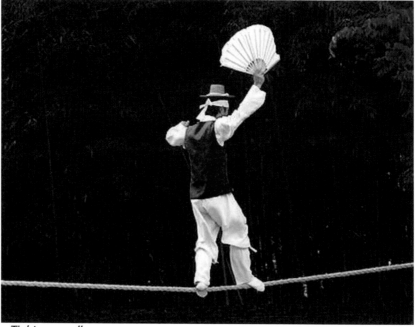

Tightrope walker

Mobility enables us to adapt, to be flexible, to go with the flow, to change course. A major concern of aging is loss of balance, leading to falls. When elderly people are afraid of falling, the tendency is to bind flow. Ironically, this makes the possibility of falling much more likely, because they are not able to accommodate to changes in weight and space. Balancing requires continuing to move, not stopping movement. We are always in the process of adjusting and balancing, but are not consciously aware of this. Try this: Stand up with your feet directly underneath you. Stand still. Now close your eyes and become aware of the gentle, subtle swaying action of stillness. If you want to challenge yourself, try this again, but start by standing on one leg with your eyes open. Notice the ongoing actions of the supporting leg and foot. Then try this with your eyes closed. Feel how holding or gripping is not a good way to maintain your balance!

A current trend in the world of fitness is an emphasis on core stability. Gyms now use special apparatus (Physioballs, Wobble Boards) that require the mover to attend to stabilizing the body while performing a variety of strengthening moves. Here we have another example of how a part has become separated from the Whole. Stability is one aspect of movement. The other side of this duality is mobility, which is equally important to the Whole of movement. The opposite of stability is not instability, but rather, mobility. The reason you use a ball to stabilize is because of its mobile nature!

Stability and mobility are intimately connected. You can't have one without the other. Strength alone will not stabilize you. Strength is a component of both stability and mobility. At the gym, it is possible to do a lot of actions, but it is not the same as working toward increasing mobility. Both mobility and stability require awareness and modulation of the body's flow. In order to balance successfully, you must have a successful balance between mobility and stability.

Exertion/Recuperation

In our culture, we operate from a work ethic. Hard work is valued. However, imbalance can occur when work is seen as separate from rest or play. The old saying, "All work and no play make Jack a dull boy", recognizes this imbalance. The work/play duality is a good example of how we compartmentalize our lives. Work is not the opposite of play, but rather its companion (and soul mate).

Work is frequently seen as necessary, serious and a requirement of life as an adult. Play is often seen as unnecessary, frivolous, and the domain of children. While this has changed to a degree from the time of the Puritans, we still adhere to this mind set. Ironically, advancements in technology were originally viewed from the perspective of increasing leisure time. Now however, how many of us are slaves to our computers, our cars, our cell phones and Blackberries? Technology took us out of the realm of manual labor and thus further away from our bodies. So rather than providing increased recuperation from labor, technology just changed how we exert ourselves!

The duality of Exertion/Recuperation is built in to the rhythm and phrasing of life. Our heart rests between beats. We sleep, we wake. We go and stop. Patterns of exertion and recuperation are the basis of rhythm. Try this: start tapping your foot and keep going until it begins to feel uncomfortable. This is a rhythm of action followed by no action, exertion of flexion of the ankle (which lifts the foot) followed by release into gravity as the foot drops. This simple rhythm is a metaphor for larger life rhythms. If you kept tapping your foot without a break, eventually you would experience fatigue – indicating that a larger rhythm was out of balance.

It is clear that we need breaks after exertions. Musicians "take five", schools schedule recess, labor unions stipulate break times. Think for a moment about the word "break". To break something is one way of creating an ending. What does it mean to say, "give me a break"? In both instances the break is an opportunity for change. The adage "a change is as good as a rest" clearly illustrates the recuperative power of change.

In fact, one man's exertion may be another man's recuperation. Like all dualities, the two are relative. For a professional tennis player, a round of tennis might not be the best recuperation. For someone who sits at a computer for several hours a day, a round of tennis could be very recuperative. Attending to the body's physical needs for a balance between exertion and recuperation is important to overall health and well-being. Although this gets lip service, the patterns of work and play still practiced in our culture are symptomatic of our disembodiment. Our culture still rewards over-exertion. Examples abound: high school athletes pushed to the point of injury, medical students working well past the point of cognitive impairment, the notion of billable hours for lawyers, the fact that overtime pays extra, etc. And while some people might regard going to the gym after work as an opportunity to recuperate, it is still referred to as "a work out". Why do we not "play in"? Here is yet another example of how language both reflects and affects the ways in which we experience movement.

Think about your own patterns of Exertion/Recuperation, both at the micro and macro level. Do you really recuperate when you take a break? Do you work and then rest, or do you work and then collapse? What type of movement do you do at work? Are you sitting or standing in one position for long periods of time? What parts of your body are most active? While recuperation does not have to be an opposite action, it does have to be a *change* of action. Someone who sits at the computer reading is not really recuperating by going home and reading the newspaper. While the sitting position and reading material may be different, the body is not really reaping the benefits of balancing the rhythm of exertion with recuperation. In this example there is a difference between rest and recuperation. Reading the newspaper after work may seem restful, but may not be real recuperation. In terms of body organization, weight support and movement rhythm (among other things), no substantive recuperative change has occurred.

Patterns of Exertion/Recuperation are phrases that establish the rhythm of our lives. A phrase is a Whole unto itself, but also part of a larger Whole. Each day has a rhythm, as does a year. Phrasing permeates the smallest discrete activities, such as how you brush your teeth, to the larger patterns that become our lives, even our civilizations (the rise and fall of the Roman Empire).
Exertion/Recuperation is the essence of the ebb and flow of the Micro/Macro in the Part/Whole theme. Note the dualities used here to describe this idea!

Ongoing exertion without recuperation is a familiar aspect of many of our lives. We call it "stress" and say we are "stressed out". We turn ourselves inside out through overexertion, leading to mental/physical meltdown. A balance between exertion and recuperation is essential to optimal living but is a challenge in today's often dis-embodied world.

Inner/Outer

All our senses, filtered through our perceptions, are bridges between our inner and outer worlds. There is an ongoing dance between the inner experience of ourselves and the outer environment with which we interact. At any moment, either can take the lead.

Our inner world includes sensations, our private thoughts and emotions. It is both our biology and our psychology. The idea of "inner" is in large part, the way in which we define ourselves. The outer world is everything that is "other", or not self. The duality of Inner/Outer is another way of languaging the theme of Self/Other.

One of the paradoxes of dis-embodiment is that, while you can't escape from yourself, you can often lose yourself. We lose ourselves through mind-altering drugs, alcohol and other addictions, and also by cutting ourselves off from bodily sensation. We lose the Whole of ourselves by over-emphasizing some parts of ourselves over other parts. While it is sometimes necessary and even fruitful to lose yourself (the aha! moment of creativity, blocking out pain to survive, a moment of spiritual transcendence) it is not possible, or even healthy, to remain out of touch with the Whole of yourself. We have all experienced occasions of deprivation during moments of extreme excitement (sleepless nights, lack of food) but we eventually must attend to the Whole of ourselves or suffer the consequences of physical and/or mental breakdown.

As with all dualities, sometimes inner is in the foreground of awareness, and sometimes outer is in the foreground. It is the ability to modulate or shift between the two (and feel how each supports the other) that promotes balance for optimal living.

Think of someone you know who seems to lack self-awareness. If someone is stuck in an outer perspective, perhaps they take on too much, can't say no, are too eager to please others at the expense of their own well-being. Or this may also be a person who comes across as superficial, lacking inner resources and empathy. Paradoxically, someone stuck in inner awareness may also come across as superficial, narcissistic and lacking in empathy. Imbalance in either direction diminishes Wholeness.

Take for example, a person who has learned to remove himself from bodily sensation in order to keep going. Fatigue, hunger, aches and pains are ignored in the face of looming deadlines. In this example, the imbalance occurs in patterns of Exertion/ Recuperation, as well as in patterns of Inner/Outer attending, and in Function/Expression. The body, in an effort to cope with unreasonable demands, begins to break down, creating imbalances in the mobility and stability of all biological systems. Muscles cramp, joints lock, the processes of breathing and digestion are compromised. All of the thematic dualities come into play, as all are interconnected. Dualities are different lenses through which to view the Whole.

Returning to the body as our basis of experience, the breathing process is a fundamental example of the two domains of inner and outer. As we inhale, we take into ourselves a part of our environment, which is then altered through our biology, and we give back a part of ourselves to the world that surrounds us. The world has changed us. We have changed the world. Poetic metaphoric descriptions of breath reflect the profundity of the Inner/Outer theme. We describe the life cycle as bounded by our first and final breaths. Things that leave us breath-less or take our breath away are of great importance. To breathe life into something is to create or revive. The power and poignancy of breath is reflected in our language.

Dualities within Wholeness

Language reflects the experience of our moving bodies. Our speaking self and our moving self are two aspects of the same self. Our capacity for language creates a uniquely human ability to analyze our experience by labeling and categorizing it. Organizing our experience into themes of duality is one way we do this. Above, we discussed four examples of dualities: Function/Expression, Stability/Mobility, Exertion/Recuperation and Inner/Outer. There are, of course, countless other possible dualities to recognize. To name a few: macro/micro perspectives, simplicity/complexity, release/control, coming/going, action/stillness, now/then, here/there, day/night, large/small, right/wrong, happy/sad, and on and on . . .

An important duality that comes into play here is the distinction between analysis and synthesis. All dualities are descriptions of two parts of a greater Whole. The process of analysis is incomplete however, until the parts are returned to the context of the Whole through the process of synthesis. Remember that language evolves from movement. We move before we speak and speaking itself is action. Conscious awareness of how movement is embedded in our language helps us to understand how movement of the body is the basis of being.

EveryBody is a speaking self and a moving self. EveryBody has two aspects of the Whole self.

Chapter 3

The Movement of Breath

The Bridge of Breath

The Rhythm of Breath

The Body of Breath

The Voice of Breath

The Anatomy of Breath

The Shape Change of Breath

Chapter 3

The Movement of Breath

"Breath is the bridge which connects life to consciousness, which unites your body to your thoughts." Thich Nhat Hanh

The Bridge of Breath

We breathe. We breathe from the moment of birth and we continue to breathe until the moment of death. It is breath that fuels the energetic processes that sustain life, and breath is the medium through which our expressive selves move out into the world. Each breath connects us to the world. Through breath, we are engaged in continuous dialogue between our inner selves and the outer world. We sigh, laugh, sob, moan, talk, sing and shout in an ongoing portrait of who we are and how we are feeling through all the moments of our life, whether we are conscious of it or not. The changing quality, depth and pattern of our breath, reveals us to others and contains the record of our past. Sharing breath bonds us in intimate relationships. To diminish breath is to diminish our ability to experience the life of the body. To expand the potential of breath is to expand the Whole of our being.

There are an astonishing number and variety of breathing practices. Some promote spiritual enlightenment and transformation. Some focus on enhancing the performance of specific skills such as singing, martial arts, weight lifting and even giving birth. All address the fundamental importance of breath. Breath "practices" acknowledge that a change in how we breathe will result in a corresponding change in our experience of life. This indicates that breathing is a powerful catalyst for life change.

The Rhythm of Breath

Like everything else, breath is defined by movement. The movement of breathing is a simple two-part phrase. We inhale; we exhale. This two-part rhythm is one of life's basic rhythms and is mirrored in many life rhythms, such as our heartbeat and our walking pattern. This biphasic rhythm is reflected even in our anatomy with its bilateral symmetry: two arms, two eyes, two sides of the brain (and so on). Breath is a cycle of movement, and, like all repetitive movement, it becomes patterned over time. Each person's baseline breath pattern is characteristic of unique activities, habits, attitudes, values, upbringing and personal history. The way one breathes becomes a part of one's personal movement signature and overlays all the obvious physiological changes in breath that must occur as we move through the day.

How we perceive the rhythm of our breath is also indicative of how we perceive parts in relationship to the Whole. Try this: take a few moments to become aware of the rhythm of your breath. Do you perceive the rhythm of your breath to be one action: beginning at the moment of inhalation and finishing with the end of exhalation? Or, does one breath have two actions – one of inhaling and another of exhaling?

Attending to breath brings our patterns to light and helps us to identify how and why these patterns serve us – or perhaps don't. Once we are aware of the rhythmic patterns of breath, we are free to explore how breath can be changed – or, more profoundly – how *we* can be changed.

The Body of Breath

The quality, depth and duration of breath can support or interfere with larger movements of the body. We know this from life experience. To "take a deep breath" can prepare us for action, as well as slow us down. Relaxation techniques rely upon awareness of, and attention to, breath. There are many philosophies about how to breathe to enhance performance, and their effectiveness is as individual as the breather. There is no one correct breathing technique. However, there are ways to breathe that are more (or less) supportive to a specific movement intention. Awareness of breath and the power it has to support our intentions is a key to full and efficient movement. Because breath is so fundamental to our moment-to-moment experience, it is easy to lose sight of its importance. Try this: take a breath. What are you aware of? Was it audible? Were you aware of movement in your chest, your shoulders, your belly? Did you breathe in through your nose or your mouth? Once you thought about your breath, were you aware of controlling it in some way or was it free and easy?

The movements of the muscles of breath cause our bodies to change shape as we breathe. On the inhalation our inner space is expanded in all three dimensions; our length, our width and our depth. The muscular actions of breathing cause our ribs to spread outward as well as lift upward as we inhale. The process of inhalation also compresses our abdominal contents, causing them to bulge outward. As we exhale, the body's inner space condenses toward center. We have more awareness of the movement of the front surface of the chest when we breathe, but we breathe into the backspace as well. Try this: A good way to experience whether or not you are breathing fully is to place one hand on your lower back and the other on your belly. Do you feel movement in both hands? It is not uncommon for the backward component of the movement of breath to be diminished. Breathing into your hands in this manner can give you more awareness of the full potential of your breath.

Becoming aware of your breath connects you to your body and thus, to yourself. This awareness of self is a first step in becoming aware of your movement.

The Voice of Breath

All vocalizing, whether public speaking, operatic singing or the cooing and babbling of a baby, depends upon the support of breath. Becoming aware of your voice and the support of breath as you speak is yet another way to become more aware of your moving self. During an aerobic workout, a common clue to the level of your exertion is whether you are too out of breath to carry on a normal conversation. When someone appears to be choking on something, we check to see if they can speak before applying the Heimlich Maneuver. Our ability to transform our thoughts into the movement of spoken language rides the flow of our breath. Try this: Recite or sing the alphabet out loud while being aware of how you are using your breath. Now try it again, but this time vocalize while inhaling. Notice the difference in the quality of sound that you produce, as well as the amount of exertion involved. This is a good example of how breath supports the action of speech.

Memorable oratory and persuasive speeches are frequently not just the words in and of themselves. What moves us is also the movement of the speaker producing the words. The power, the rhythm, the intonation and vocal articulation are the result of movement. Even twangs or accents result from the movement patterning of speech. Vocal recognition is the recognition of the movements of speech. A cornerstone of an actor's training is learning to control and modulate movement of the vocal apparatus. Breath, as the bridge between our inner and outer worlds, supports how we are able to express our thoughts and interact with others via spoken language.

The Anatomy of Breath

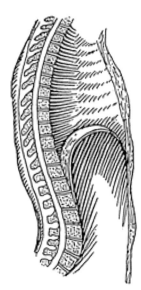

Just a brief review of basic breathing anatomy can hint at the actual complexity of this deceptively simple rhythm of life.

The primary mover of breath is a unique muscle called the Thoracic Diaphragm. The word 'diaphragm' is used to describe any membrane or partition that separates one thing from another, and that vibrates and/or transmits light, energy or fluids across itself. We have many different types of diaphragms within our body, from the lens of the eye to the floor of the pelvis.

Lateral view of the dome shape of the Diaphragm

The muscle of breath is the Thoracic Diaphragm. It is the structure that forms the ceiling of the abdominal cavity and the floor of the chest cavity, thus separating the structure of our inner volume. It also marks the difference between our upper and lower body. The Thoracic Diaphragm is shaped like a lopsided mushroom, higher on the right side due to the size and position of the liver. The cap of the mushroom fills the circumference of the rib cage and is moved up and down by the action of the stem of the mushroom (two extensions of muscle tissue called the crura) which is attached to the front surface of the lower spine. Inhalation results from the crura contracting to pull the cap downward, creating a vacuum in the thorax so that air can then rush in to fill our lungs. On the exhale, the crura relax and the cap recoils upward, pushing air out of the lungs.

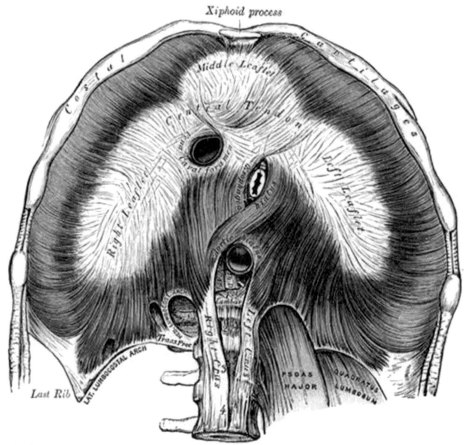

Thoracic diaphragm seen from below, with crura attached to spine

The Thoracic Diaphragm is intimately connected with our deepest abdominal muscle, the Transversalis. This muscle, which can be envisioned as an internal cummerbund, decreases the circumference of the waist when it contracts. The Transversalis (aka Transversus Abdominus) can be viewed as a muscle of self expression, because it gets noticeably sore after extreme exhalations or expulsions. Laughing, sobbing, shouting, vomiting and coughing are the domain of the Transversalis, adding power as needed to the relaxation phase of the Thoracic Diaphragm. Try this: Place your hands above your belly button and force the air out quickly. The action your feel under your hands is the Transversalis at work.

The lifting and lowering action of the Diaphragm reiterates the vertical nature of our upright form. The Thoracic Diaphragm is located at the body's core and it shares intimate relationships with other muscles of core support such as the Quadratus Lumborum and the Iliopsoas. These deep muscles working harmoniously together support the connection between our upper and lower body. Ligaments of the Diaphragm arch over the Quadratus Lumborum – the muscle that knits together the back of the lower ribs with the top of the pelvis. Notice that this too is a bridge between the upper and lower body. Therefore, our breathing connects the functional and expressive mobility of our upper and lower bodies.

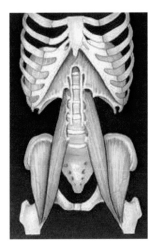

The Thoracic Diaphragm shares the attachment of its contractile portion (the crura) with the upper portion of the Iliopsoas muscle on the front (anterior surface) of the lumbar spine. The Iliopsoas is our deepest and most efficient flexor of the hip because of its attachments to the spine and upper leg. It is easier to engage the Iliopsoas for hip flexion during an exhale, when the Thoracic Diaphragm is moving upward during the relaxation phase and pressure is no longer bulging the lower abdomen.

Interrelationship of Iliopsoas and Thoracic Diaphragm

Important structures of other body systems penetrate the Thoracic Diaphragm. The aorta and blood vessels of the circulatory system, the lymphatic system, the esophagus, and nerves are all affected by, and affect breathing. It is not an exaggeration to say that all life processes are affected by and affect breathing. For example, when we have a case of the hic-ups, our normal breath rhythm is interrupted, which can become annoying and distract us from our activities. Awareness of breath can help reduce stress. It can also increase energy and multiple other things as well! The advice to "take a deep breath" speaks to our understanding of how breath supports and serves us.

The Shape Change of Breath

Breath is a vital part of the experience of Shape Flow, that ongoing conversation of the body with itself. As first addressed in Chapter 1, Shape Flow serves the function of self-monitoring. Weight shifts, adjustments in posture, moments of self touch as you rub a sore spot or brush hair out of your face, serve to keep us connected to ourselves throughout the day. Our breath too reflects the process of Shape Flow. While some Shape Flow breath patterns can be distracting (sighing or yawning), too little Shape Flow and diminished breath deadens self-awareness.

Experience of breath is an essential experience of self and as such it is a vital part of the self-monitoring process. We prepare with the Shape Flow of breath and recuperate with the Shape Flow of breath. No matter what our mood is, our breathing reflects our state of being. Subsequently, breath can also be used to elicit particular states of being. Your breathing can relax you or energize you. It can serve to sustain you or galvanize you. Try this: Breathe in. Become aware of your sensations. If your inner volume were a balloon, how would the balloon change shape? Do you feel your ribs moving? Your belly? What happens when you release the air?

Because breathing is largely an involuntary process, we are often not aware of possible patterns of breathing which are restricting our full potential to move, to feel, to respond, to be. For example, a young girl taking ballet lessons may unconsciously make her breathing small and shallow in order to experience herself as smaller and thinner. This pattern can carry over into all aspects of daily life, limiting access to full breath potential. Ironically, while she may feel thinner, the expression of her dancing is diminished. Coming into conscious awareness of our breathing promotes self-awareness, and gives us the benefit of more ease and energy.

Throughout our life: we breathe deeply, our breath is bated, we hold our breath, we whisper and shout, sing and cry, blow out the candles on a cake, blow kisses, give speeches, sigh, moan, babble, suck it in and let it out. The power of breath is profound. Breath is a hallmark of human experience – it is synonymous with life.

Awareness of breath supports movement. Breath supports our everyday functional activities, our athletic pursuits, our creative expression, our personal interactions. Breath literally supports EveryBody in all aspects of life.

Chapter 4

Weight in All its Many Guises

Weight as Basic Experience

The Weight Obsession

Weight Sensing – The Bond of Weight and Flow

Supporting Our Weight – Active or Passive

Another Duality – Our Weight in Relationship to the Earth

Moving Our Weight Through Space

Our Weight is Us

Chapter 4

Weight in All its Many Guises

*"Weight is **what** we move." Laura Cox*

Weight as Basic Experience

One of the primary ways in which we experience ourselves is through the experience of our body's weight. We have mass and we exist in a world subject to the laws of gravity. Gravity is what literally connects us to the world. Without gravity, we would become untethered from the Earth. Our experience of weight (our relationship to gravity) is so basic to the essence of being human that we take it for granted. Weight is so fundamental that it becomes conflated with abstractions of other aspects of human experience. Look at some of the many ways we use the word "weight". We feel the weight of our responsibilities. We weigh our options to make a decision. We put our weight behind something we truly believe in. We throw our weight around to influence others. Carrying the weight can be a burden both emotionally and physically. Just as the patterns of our flow define us, our sense of weight too, is fundamental to our sense of self.

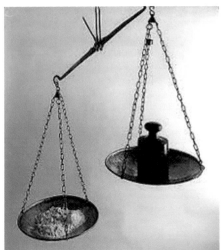

Old fashioned balance scales

The Weight Obsession

There is an obsession in our modern culture with weight in its guise of poundage and how our weight in pounds is a symbol of our relative health or appearance. Although issues of fashion and obesity are clearly connected to the Function/Expression of weight, we are not going to specifically address this aspect of weight here. The exaggerated emphasis on the importance of how much one weighs is one symptom of a lack of Whole body awareness. We compartmentalize

35

the component of over-weight or under-weight as if it represented the totality of health and well-being. This obsession with weight is indicative of the cultural pattern of mistaking a part for the Whole. Becoming more conscious of the totality of your physical being can result in more balance among all considerations related to wellness and may also lead to a more optimal weight as measured by a scale.

Weight Sensing – The Bond of Weight and Flow

Have you ever noticed athletes before a competition, or performers before a show? It is common to see actions of weight sensing such as bouncing, pulsing, rocking, jiggling or shaking. These actions help the performers to connect to themselves as preparation for the event to come. Weight sensing helps them to center and ground themselves. Try this: gently bounce up and down. Notice as you bounce, that you actively lift and then let go to drop. In other words, you activate your weight to lift and then release your weight, yielding to gravity as you drop. Slow the bounce down, making sure that you really allow your weight to collapse when you drop. Feel the difference between the active (lift) and passive (release) roles of weight in the bounce. Compare the sensation of this full release of weight to a bounce in which you hold on to weight while binding your flow. For example, when children really have to go to the bathroom, they never really release their weight in the bouncing action. We can imagine what would happen if they did!

The bi-phasic action of activating and "passivating" the weight of our bodies is related to how we Mobilize/Stabilize. Releasing our weight allows us to connect to our base of support. This connection is the stable platform from which we can efficiently mobilize. Allowing weight to become passive through the process of release is the first step in activating weight to push away from support.

The bouncing action of weight sensing described above is also connected to the concept of Shape Flow discussed earlier in Chapter 1. Just like flow, weight underlies our sense of self. Weight and flow are fundamentally connected through our movement. Our body's weight rides the flow as we mobilize to activate the weight or allow it to "give in" to gravity. In both cases weight is linked to the ongoing progression of flow. The union of weight and flow contributes to our conscious awareness as independent beings capable of action. Flow connects us to the universal. Weight connects us to the personal. We create ourselves through the patterns of our movement. "I" act and am carried forward on the continuing flow of my existence.

Weight sensing also promotes balance between Inner/Outer and Exertion/Recuperation. In preparation for an event, an athlete uses weight sensing to maintain awareness of the external goal he is moving toward (Outer) while connecting to himself in the present moment (Inner). At the end of the day, when you lie down to sleep, the ability to release your flow and weight is as crucial to the recuperation of a good night's sleep as a good mattress.

Many people enjoy swings, slides, roller coasters and other activities that provide pleasurable sensations of weight and flow. Babies love to be bounced and love to bounce themselves. People use rocking chairs and rocking actions to both energize and soothe themselves. We rock the cradle and we "rock out" to Rock music. Sensations of weight and flow connect us to ourselves and to one another.

Supporting our Weight – Active or Passive

Become aware of how are you currently supporting your weight. If you are seated, is your weight equally supported on both sides? Are both feet on the floor or is one leg crossed? If your leg is crossed, that leg is actually being supported by the other leg underneath it. If your feet are on the floor, they too are part of the support team. Weight support occurs throughout the body. When sitting in a chair, as you adjust your position, you are changing how your weight is supported. If your chair is at a table or desk, you can sit upright with your back not resting on the chair. Or you can lean back against the chair for support. You can also lean forward, placing your elbows on the table to support the weight of the head in your hand. In the process of weight support, weight can be either active or passive. Try this: Sit with an elbow resting on a table and really let your head rest on your hand. In resting, you are letting your head be propped up by your hand and arm. Take a moment to feel the weight of your heavy head. In this case, the weight of your head is passive and if someone knocked your arm out from under your head, you would have to actively engage weight support to avoid abruptly dropping your head.

We need to have access to both the active and passive aspects of our weight experience. For instance, you settle into an easy chair to relax, allowing your body to become heavy. Really "letting go" involves letting our weight become passive. Then, you hear a crash in the next room and you activate your weight in preparation for an appropriate response. The ability to mobilize in response is an active use of weight.

Be aware however, that too much passivity, or too much activity, can be immobilizing. As in all dualities, harmony is achieved by balance between both sides. In the above example, the longer you hang out in your easy chair, the harder it may be to find both the motivation and physical strength to get up! It is also true that too much activation without recuperation can be immobilizing. Ideas about good posture can lead to a rigid vertical stance in which weight and flow are actively held by muscle work. In this case, over-activation of weight support is inefficient and can lead to pain and fatigue.

Become aware of how you support your weight. When standing in line at the grocery store, do you let your weight become passive by sinking into one hip, locking your knees or collapsing your chest? These passive positions will not support you for long without discomfort. We can most efficiently support our weight through subtle ongoing active change. The next time you find yourself standing in line for something, allow yourself to consciously engage in recuperation through ongoing active weight adjustments.

Another Duality – Our Weight in Relationship to the Earth

Another aspect to the experience of gravity is counterthrust. You may recall that one of Isaac Newton's laws of motion states that for every action there is an equal and opposite reaction (balance). The downward direction of our weight due to gravity is balanced by an equal upward thrust from the earth, which supports us and assists us with activating our weight. Although we are not generally aware of this, the earth literally gives us a boost! The next time you are standing in line for a while, become aware of, and connect to, the resilient upward thrust from the earth that supports you and allows you to simultaneously mobilize and stabilize as you wait. This is an active, energetic connection to your weight, rather than a passive propping of body parts.

Just as our weight exists in relationship to the earth, active and passive weight also exist in relationship to each other. Seemingly a paradox, in order to effectively activate your weight, you must first yield to gravity (passive weight) which allows your weight to be fully supported by the earth. This is the process of grounding your weight. The term "grounding" becomes a metaphor for laying the foundation for knowledge and understanding. For instance, an educational pamphlet might state, "Every child needs a good grounding in both the arts and sciences".

From a grounded position of support, weight can then be activated most efficiently. This activation is the movement of pushing. Push patterns are primary foundational patterns of human movement. As discussed in Chapter 2 and throughout the text, we reference these primary movement patterns in our language. Describing someone as pushy is a direct link to our embodied experience.

Moving our Weight Through Space

There are many complex life forms that don't travel through space. Trees don't locomote, and other species plant themselves in one spot, where they remain for the duration of their lives. Moving through space is one of the things that characterize human beings. When we travel from one spot to another, we are mobilizing our weight.

How does this happen? While it is possible to move the weight of one part of the body without traveling, in order to travel, the center of our weight must shift. We can march in place and not go anywhere. When our marching takes us someplace, it is because we have engaged our center of weight. What and where is the center of body weight? For the purpose of understanding human movement, the terms center of weight, center of gravity and center of mass are indistinguishable. In the body, the center of gravity is the location where weight or mass is most concentrated. Generally, in the typical upright stance of an adult, this point is located in the pelvis. When the center of gravity moves beyond the base of support, the body as a Whole will shift to a new location in space. Walking results from the propulsion of our center of weight through space. The role of the legs is to catch, support and transfer the weight center as we travel from one place to another.

In order to travel (locomote), we have to shift our weight. Walking is not simply a pattern of flexion and extension of the legs. Every step we take is a postural shift that involves the pelvis, which mobilizes our center of weight. The action of the legs supports the shift of the pelvis as we walk. The fact that the pelvis is mobile while also having to support weight makes it vital in postural action and locomotion. An awareness and understanding of how the pelvis functions is important for efficiently moving through space and maintaining the ability to move fully and freely throughout the course of one's life. Lower back pain, which is rampant in our culture, is often a direct result of diminished pelvic function in its role of weight support and movement.

Unfortunately, other associations with movement of the pelvis override this simple fact. We have different associations with different parts of the body. Our upper body, as the home of both our heads and our hearts, is associated with thinking and feeling. The lower body, as the home of our organs of procreation and elimination, carries different cultural baggage. The biological functions of the pelvis frequently overshadow the vital role the pelvis plays in moving us through space. As a result, our ability to locomote can be hampered. We associate pelvic movement with sexual expression and the biological process of elimination to the detriment of the functional aspect of weight shift. We focus on a part of pelvic function rather than the Wholeness of movement potential. This is further complicated by advancements in technology that reduce our need to move and take us away from conscious awareness of Whole body movement.

Moving our weight through space is an ongoing process between mobilizing and stabilizing. This is the process of balance, and balance is dynamic. In Chapter 2, we noted the common misperception that the opposite of mobility is immobility and the opposite of stability is instability. In reality, mobility and stability create a duet. Each needs the other to complete the partnership. Try this again: stand completely still. You will soon become aware that absolute stillness is impossible. Now stand on one foot. Notice how you maintain your balance. Now close your eyes while standing on one foot. This experience illustrates the dynamic nature of ongoing balance. It also exemplifies the continuity between Inner/Outer. You probably noticed that it was more difficult to balance when you closed your eyes, because we use vision as an external cue to help stabilize us.

Another way in which we stabilize is through the process of counter-balance. When we move our weight, one of two things will happen. We will either move through space (fall over or locomote) or counter-balance one weight shift with another in order to maintain our base of support. Try this: Start standing with your weight equally balanced on both feet. Reach to one side. Continue to reach and notice how your weight shifts. If you reach even further, how do you counter-balance in order to keep from falling? Did you notice how the opposite side of your body became involved in a shift to the other direction?

Our Weight is Us

We experience ourselves through the experience of our weight. Our weight is our tangible physical essence and fundamental to our individuality. The primacy of our weight experience is at the core of our obsession with how much we weigh and what we believe our weight reveals about us. We equate weight with Self. This is why we may perceive someone who is over-weight as someone who lacks self-control. The reality is there are multiple factors at play, including genetic predisposition and the environment.

When we manifest our will, our intention in the world, we move our weight. We use the term weight to suggest value, significance and seriousness. We weigh in on a matter when we want our opinion to count. We give more weight to advice from someone we respect. Our experience of our weight is directly related to our sense of presence in the world, and we make an impact on the world through asserting our weight.

The experience of weight is profound. It connects us to ourselves and connects us to the world. It is a foundation from which EveryBody expresses themselves in the world.

Chapter 5

Moving the Parts/Moving the Whole

Gesture/Posture – Part/Whole

Multi-Part Harmony

Dynamic Alignment

Our Architectural Support: The Skeleton

Our Voluminous 3D Form

Chapter 5

Moving The Parts / Moving The Whole

"The whole is more than the sum of its parts." Aristotle

To appreciate the beauty and complexity of the body in motion, think of an analogy to a symphonic score. Each individual instrument has its own specific part and is sometimes emphasized (a climactic cymbal crash, for example). All the instrumental parts working together, coming in and out at various times and blending their individual voices, create the Whole of the musical composition. Our body parts, moving together in coordinated patterns, create the Whole of the synergy of movement.

Gesture/Posture – Part/Whole

It is possible to move parts of our body in isolation. We do it all the time. We nod our head, we wave our hand, we tap our foot. All of these isolated actions are gestures. A gestural change is a change in the relationship of a part of the body with the Whole. A postural change produces a change of the Whole body. You are moving posturally when you shift your weight to a new position while sitting or standing in line. You haven't gone anywhere, but you have made a postural shift. Try this: sitting on your chair, fold your arms across you chest. This action did not require a postural shift of weight, so it was an upper body gestural change. Now shift your body's weight, moving you into a new position. Did you notice the difference? A change of the Whole expresses something different from a change of a part.

Once again, there are functional as well as expressive attributes to any change. Imagine an adult and a child playing a board game together. The adult is more likely to move a game piece as a gesture, while the child is more likely to move posturally as he plays the game. Functionally, the adult has learned to achieve a greater level of differentiation in movement. Also, the adult is more aware that the game is only a part of the activities of the day. The child, however, is more fully invested in the play, which is revealed in a greater number of postural shifts when compared with the adult. He is committed to the moment in a different way than the adult is, reflecting a different relationship of part to the Whole.

Gestures and postures are not mutually exclusive actions. A gesture can lead us into a new posture, or a posture can resolve itself into a gesture. Try this: start with the gesture of raising your hand, as if you are in a classroom setting. Now, really try to get the teacher's attention by extending the gesture through the torso until you feel the postural change. Note the shift in intensity and attitude. To feel the change that happens when a posture segues into a gesture, now try this: start from an upright sitting posture, allow your weight to collapse passively and then let the head fall toward the chest at the end. Can you feel how this final gesture of the head is the result of the postural change? When posture and gesture merge together within a movement expression, the meaningfulness of the movement intensifies. A posture/gesture merger indicates a committed intention on the part of the mover.

Multi-Part Harmony

In considering human movement however, we tend to think of the body as a collection of parts, and attend to the parts in isolation. For example, traditional models of good posture view the body in an upright standing position, with blocks of body parts (head, ribcage, pelvis) stacked one on top of another aligned with gravity. But what happens when the body begins to move or maintain an off-vertical position? The block model does not take into consideration the relationship of the parts to each other. But, in fact, just as in a symphony, the parts of our bodies are designed to move harmoniously in complex phrases.

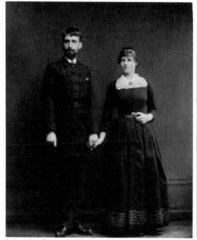 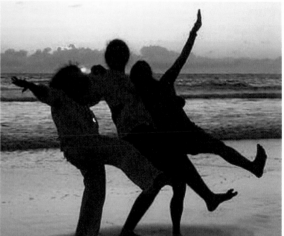

Vertical upright posture   *Off vertical posture*

The following is an example of how we too frequently separate the parts from the Whole. At the gym a physical trainer may tell you to make sure that the knee of your weight-bearing leg is aligned over your ankle when performing a lunge. This directive focuses on the lunge **position**, not the **action** of lunging. The action of a lunge is a weight shift, which comes from the center of the body. It is not simply a bend of the knee. Rather than focusing on the position of parts (knee to ankle), it is important to address the changing relationship of parts as they move. Awareness of the movement **process** rather than the end **position** is essential in preventing potential damage to the knee. Awareness of the parts of the body in relation to the Whole body is fundamental in optimizing physical function and promoting functional longevity.

The body as a Whole is made up of a multitude of different parts. All of these parts move in relationship to the other parts. We have many ways to categorize/identify the parts of the body. Traditional anatomical models differentiate body parts by structure, physiological models differentiate body parts through functional systems: respiratory, digestive, circulatory, etc. The science of medicine identifies specializations based on both parts and function. We go to a dentist in one case, an internist in another. Western medicine emphasizes differentiating the parts from the Whole, whereas Eastern medicine places more value on treating the part in the context of the Whole. Today we are seeing the benefit of connecting these two world-views. While it can be beneficial to identify a problem through a part, it is obvious that a problem with a part of the body causes problems with the Whole. Ask anyone who has had a toothache. Categorizing the body through parts and systems is a theoretical construct that helps us to organize and analyze, but in reality the body is one organic entity in which the parts are seamlessly interwoven. In fact, one part that we identify is labeled connective tissue. Connective tissue is named for its function. It is the fabric that knits all of our inner and outer parts together to form a cohesive Whole. Connective tissue permeates and both defines and unifies all structures of the body from deep within our core to the outermost layer of skin.

Although it is possible to emphasize the action of one body part, even an isolated gesture causes a change in the relationship among the parts of the Whole body. Try this: turn your head. Your visual field changes, along with the relationships of your cervical vertebrae and skull, upper body muscles, and even a subtle shift in weight distribution. When a change occurs in any part of the body, the Whole body changes in response. This is the Principle of Dynamic Alignment.

Dynamic Alignment

Dynamic Alignment is awareness of the ongoing relationship among our parts as we move through the world. We are always in a process of change (which is dynamic) and we are always in some pattern of relationship of parts (alignment). We are in relationship to the parts of ourselves, and we ourselves are in relationship with the world and beyond. The architecture of our body exists harmoniously within the larger context of the architecture of space. Thus the concept of alignment can be seen from a macro perspective of the alignment of the stars and the planets, to a more micro perspective of the alignment of the spine, describing someone's posture.

We have more than 200 bones, several hundred muscles, and a multitude of other parts including organs, tendons, ligaments, blood vessels, etc. The larger movement of our bodies as Wholes is accomplished through the micro movements of smaller parts of us. The movement of chemicals through our blood stream, the electrochemical firing of nerves, the secretion of enzymes, peristalsis, heartbeat and breath, are all movements that contribute to moving our body as a Whole.

Most of our biological functions are generally not under our conscious control. A part that we do control, even though we are not always aware of it, is the movement of our musculoskeletal system.

The movement of the musculoskeletal system results from the following sequence of events: an electrochemical message from the nervous system (conscious or unconscious in response to stimulus) is sent to the muscles, which contract to pull on bones, creating a change in the relationship of the bones at their joints.

Joints are the place where bones meet, thus joints are where musculoskeletal movement happens. Our bones have many shapes and sizes, so their connections vary in structure. These structural differences produce different types of action, ranges and degrees of movement through space. Most joint actions result in motion either toward or away from our body. Interestingly, joint actions are identified dualistically in pairs of opposite actions: flexion/extension, abduction/adduction, inward/outward rotation, right/left rotation, right/left lateral flexion. These opposite joint actions are linked to spatial opposition relative to the body. For example, actions of abduction move the limbs sideways away from the body. Adduction is the opposite action, in which the limbs move sideways towards from the body. Jumping Jacks are a perfect illustration of the spatial opposition of abduction and adduction.

Remember, if a part changes, the Whole changes. Not only do the bones and joints change relationship, all of our body contents change relationship as well. Movement of the musculoskeletal system results in movement of the organs and other tissues making up our Whole. This movement of the contents of our body container is necessary for our health and well-being. Prolonged immobility not only contributes to deterioration of the muscles and joints, it also adversely affects other body systems such as the circulatory system, the lymphatic system, and the digestive system.

Movement is always a change relationship. For example, when you use one hand to pick up a weight, you are not just isolating a contraction of the biceps muscle to flex the elbow. Muscles of the hand and forearm are activated to grasp and hold the weight while you are also stabilizing the muscles of your shoulder and core to minimize unwanted actions. And don't forget you are also breathing, so the muscle of the Thoracic Diaphragm is moving. All movement is a dance between what is mobile and what is stable.

Muscles work synergistically together in groups. The principle of synergy is that the Whole is greater than the sum of its parts. The synergistic relationships among muscles are what allow us to move most efficiently. Because muscles work together, they have different roles depending on the movement situation. In one instance, a muscle may be called upon to be the prime mover. In another, this same muscle may be recruited to assist a prime mover. In still another situation, the same muscle may act as a stabilizer by resisting the action of yet another muscle. The synergistic actions of muscle groups are referred to as kinetic chains.

Kinetic chains are patterned at the subconscious level. We do not have to think about the individual actions of each muscle involved in a sequence. Try this: Stand up from your chair and then sit back down. Are you able to identify the series of muscles involved in accomplishing this sequence? No. Remember our earlier example of putting on your socks? If you had to think about patterning the muscles to move all the joints involved in movement, it would take too long and is obviously inefficient.

While it is impossible to be consciously aware of every single action of every single muscle all the time, we can re-pattern kinetic chains to move more efficiently. One way of doing this is to visualize our anatomy. By visualizing relationships in skeletal anatomy, we can optimize Dynamic Alignment. For example, you would not teach a child to ride a bike or throw a ball only by telling him how to do it. You both tell him and demonstrate the movement. A large part of our motor learning results from visual cues followed by the physical experience of practice. A clear image of how the body is connected both supports and enhances physical practice. Like the song,

> *Toe bones connected to your foot bones*
> *Foot bones connected to your ankle bone*
> *Ankle bone connected to your leg bone*

And so on . . .sung with greater or lesser anatomical accuracy!

One way we compartmentalize our parts is in how we identify chronic patterns of pain and disfunction. For example, concern over Carpal Tunnel Syndrome focuses on the isolated gestural action of the wrist. Even ergonomic interventions related to chair and keyboard changes will have limited success if the mover does not make the Whole body postural changes that will relieve the symptomatic wrist pain. The action of the hand does not stop at the wrist. It continues through the forearm, upper arm, shoulder blade and is supported by the spine. In other words, the parts connect to the Whole.

The example above reflects an even larger way in which we compartmentalize. Contemporary culture has created a work environment in which the exertion of repetitive actions is not balanced by other actions. The environment promotes imbalance leading to chronic pain. Carpal Tunnel Syndrome is not only about relationships among body parts, it also reflects imbalance in the relationships of the parts of the individual's life. In a sense, Carpal Tunnel Syndrome may be seen not only as a breakdown in the function of the wrist (microanalysis), but also a breakdown in the larger patterns of our lives (macroanalysis).

Our Architectural Support: The Skeleton

To experience optimal movement patterning, we look to the body's architecture. We all recognize the human form in our vertical stance and bilateral symmetry. We are not goldfish or giraffes! Just as any animal's form dictates its movement, our particular form determines how we move. Our upper and lower bodies share similarities. We have two legs and two arms. We have ten toes and ten fingers. However, the evolution of our form into our present upright stance has resulted in (and allows for) specialized differences between our upper and lower bodies. The patterns of our movement arise from the relationships between our upper and lower body; our right and left sides; our front and back. The basic structural frame of the human form is the skeleton.

A fundamental way that we categorize the parts of our bodies is in a simple dualistic division: front and back, right and left, upper and lower. One of the ways in which the upper is different from the lower body is in terms of the Stability/Mobility relationship. Our limb bones are attached to other bones, which form a girdle connecting the limbs to the core. In the upper body, the arms connect to the shoulder girdle, in the lower body the legs connect to the pelvic girdle.

The upper body is designed for tremendous mobility and independent action of the arms. The shoulder girdle is comprised of the clavicles (collar bones) and scapulae (shoulder blades). While we identify a girdle as a continuous loop, the shoulder blades themselves do not connect directly to each other or to the spine, thus increasing upper body mobility and allowing for differentiation in the movement of the right and left arm. In fact, the shoulder blades freely float within the muscular structure of the back.

In contrast, the lower body is designed for stability in its role of weight transfer and support. The legs connect to the pelvic girdle, which includes a direct connection to the spine. Unlike the shoulder girdle, the pelvic girdle is a continuous bony structure that moves as a Whole, contributing to its ability to support and stabilize our movement.

Our skeleton supports us just as the struts, beams and framing support buildings. Our bones are our architectural infrastructure. Identifying boney relationships helps us to organize all of our parts into a connected Whole. Boney landmarks map the body and literally help to make it navigable. Movement can be thought of as a journey from here to there. Just knowing where you should end up is no guarantee that you will take the best route. Like landmarks in our landscapes, boney landmarks are notable aspects of individual bones or single bones. Just as the ability to read a map helps you get to your destination, knowledge of your bones can help guide your movement.

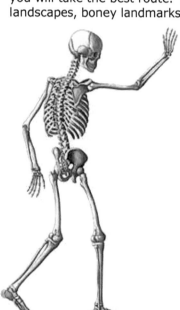

In the lunge example cited earlier, the foot is the support and the pelvis is in motion as the weight shifts to the lunging leg. We can bring the parts into relationship by experiencing the connection between the boney landmarks of the heel bone (Calcaneus) and the sit bone (Ischial Tuberosity) of the lunging leg and pelvis. Maintaining a connection between the heel and sit bone while weight shifting is just one of many possible connections that can be identified to help in organizing the journey of our movement. Try this: the next time you have trouble opening the lid of a jar, visualize the connection between your hand and your shoulder (specifically the shoulder blade, or scapula). Note that awareness of this connection can facilitate the action.

48

In another example, we can connect our upper and lower body through awareness of the opposite ends of the spine. The spine as a Whole is the boney support that connects the upper and lower body. This is the Head/Tail Connection (Skull/Coccyx). When your mother told you to "stand up straight" she was telling you to lengthen the relationship between the two ends of your spine to optimize your posture. The spine is an amazing structure. Twenty-four individual vertebral bones, plus the Sacrum and the Coccyx (tailbone) form the spine. The architecture of the spine is characterized by four distinct balancing curves. When we are born, we have just one curve. This is the familiar fetal ball shape. As we learn to support the weight of our head, the Cervical curve develops. Later, as we come to sitting and support our weight through the pelvis, the Lumbar curve develops. The ongoing necessity to both stabilize and mobilize our weight is what gives our spine its dynamic form. In essence, we create our own spinal architecture.

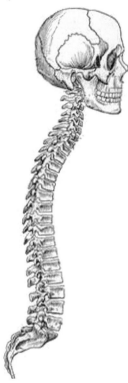

Curves of spine

The head balances on top of the seven vertebral bones called the Cervical Spine (C1-C7). The forward cervical curve changes to a backward curve in the Thoracic Spine, which supports our twelve pairs of ribs (T1-T12). The thoracic curve changes to a forward curve in the Lumbar Spine (L1-L5). The last lumbar vertebra rests on the Sacrum, a triangular bone comprised of fused vertebrae that curves backward like a scoop to complete the back of the pelvic bowl. Hanging below and continuing the sacral curve is the Coccyx, or tailbone. Each portion of the spine has a distinctive function and design. All the myriad discreet motions between and among all of the vertebrae and their discs, together create the synergy that is spinal movement. Awareness of the relationship between the two ends of our spine, the Skull and the Coccyx, can enhance the synergy of all the moveable parts in between that form the Wholeness of our upper and lower body.

The Head/Tail Connection is an example of one possible relationship between the upper and lower body. The spine is a primary skeletal structure that establishes the up and down of our upright form in relation to gravity. The spine also, as our up and down axis, establishes the midline of our bilateral symmetry, determining the right and left sides of our body. Our "sidedness" is an obvious physical fact and one that we learn to take for granted. Right or left handed-ness is related to sides of the brain, which is also connected to dominant eye, and on and on. Try this: Point your index finger up to the sky and fully extend your arm in front of you while focusing on an object in the distance. Alternate closing one eye and then the other. Notice that your field of vision has shifted. Just as your right or left hand is your dominant hand, you also have a dominant eye connected to one side of the brain. The two sides are opposite, but interdependent, and together create the Whole.

How our opposite sides connect is also evident in the way we walk, opposite arm to leg. It is possible to walk with limp arms or, like Frankenstein's monster, to walk with the same side arm and leg moving simultaneously. But the way we are wired to walk most efficiently is using leg and arm opposition.

We have a front and a back, but we are generally more aware of our front side. This is mainly due to the location of our face, particularly our eyes, and the fact that our joints flex to carry us in a forward direction. Back pain is often related to a misalignment of the pelvis, causing a swayback posture. In this alignment, the bowl of the pelvis is tipped forward. If the pelvic bowl were filled with soup, the soup would spill onto your feet. In this example, connecting two specific boney landmarks can promote balance between the front and back of the body. Try this: Stand up and place one hand on the Xiphoid Process (lowest point of the breastbone) and place the other hand on the Pubic Symphysis (boney landmark on the front surface of the pelvis approximately eight inches below the belly button). By rocking the pelvis forward and back, you can experience how the distance between these two points changes. Note the relationship between the swayback position of the Lumbar Spine and the increased distance between these two points. Perhaps use the image of zipping up the fly of your pants to bring these two boney landmarks into optimal relationship. Prescriptions for strengthening the abdominal muscles as a cure for back pain are based in part on facilitating the Wholeness of the front and back of the body. However, focusing on muscle action alone is not the solution. It is just one small piece of a greater connected Whole.

Our Voluminous 3D Form

A primary consideration for connecting our parts into an integrated Whole is the awareness of our body as a three-dimensional form. For instance, lower back pain is often perceived as occurring on the back surface of the body. However, looking at a three-dimensional model of the spine in anatomical relationship reveals that the low back (our Lumbar Spine) is actually closer to the center of the body. Connecting through the depth of our front/back volume allows us to access the full support of the body.

We are three-dimensional bodies operating in a three-dimensional environment. This fact is often ignored in traditional models of physical therapy, sports coaching and fitness. These models tend to emphasize two-dimensional isolated actions of single joints. This is not very helpful in the context of more complex full-bodied movement sequences. For example, coaching a golf swing requires an understanding of the complex three dimensional and ever-changing relationships between the upper and lower body. Is the golfer accessing an effective Head/Tail Connection while grounding through the Heel/Sit bone Connection while organizing the Hand/Scapula (shoulder blade) Connection? Attending to these and other boney connections is a direct and concise way of tapping into the complexity of the underlying muscular kinetic chains. Thinking at the level of the bone clarifies the patterning of the muscular and the nervous systems, which operate below the conscious level.

If we isolate parts, or leave parts out, we have less access to the Wholeness of self. The parts of our bodies are in continual interchanging relationships, creating EveryBody's dynamic Whole.

Chapter 6

Moving the Whole / Moving the Parts

Our Development: The Support of Underlying Patterns

Principles of Development

Core/Distal Patterning

Head/Tail Patterning (Spinal)

Upper/Lower Patterning (Homologous)

Right/Left Patterning (Homolateral)

Cross-Lateral Patterning

Re-patterning Movement

Chapter 6

Moving the Whole/Moving the Parts

*"To live is not merely to breathe; it is to act; it is to make use of our organs, senses, faculties – of all those **parts** of ourselves which give us the feeling of existence"*
Jean-Jacques Rousseau

Our Development: The Support of Underlying Patterns

Our evolution and development has led to our present form – including our upright stance, opposable thumbs, large brain, and the predominance of our visual sense over our other senses. Even many of our contemporary ailments, from back pain to knee problems, can be seen, in part, as byproducts of how our form evolved.

Built into the design of human beings are specific underlying movement patterns that support relationships among our parts. Starting from basic reflexes and inborn movement responses, we are hard-wired for movement patterns that support our survival. For example, remember the last time you started to fall asleep while sitting up and felt your head snap upright, returning to vertical position? This righting response is part of our internal wiring which underlies other patterns related to our survival from infancy onward, such as nursing and coming to standing as a bipedal individual. Unlike other mammals that are born with an almost immediate ability to support their weight and then run away from danger, the human infant goes through a long process of motor development.

This developmental process, which unrolls in a patterned sequence, solidifies and is solidified by, movement. As babies, we learn to first support our head, then roll over, then come to sitting, then crawl, then stand, then walk. Parents see these steps as important developmental milestones. Going through the process of motor development is fundamental to the creation of ourselves as individual personalities and also identifies us as human. The process is necessary to achieve skill and mastery of ourselves as movers. Through this movement progression we establish ourselves as the active agent of our own existence.

The progression of our development occurs in identifiable patterns. These patterns play out in sequence, but are also nuanced by individual variation. This is why one child walks at nine months while another walks at thirteen months. The clear pattern and progression of movement development is characterized by specific relationships among the parts of our human form. Our form, with its vertical upright stance and bilateral symmetry, is organized through relationships among upper and lower body, right and left sides of the body, front and back, core and periphery.

Principles of Development

It is important to understand some basic principles of development. Perhaps the most essential of these is that development is an ongoing building process. We sit before we stand, standing precedes walking and gross motor skills precede fine motor skills. Early skills support skills that develop later. A pattern of developmental progression is seen in all aspects of life, from the development of an individual child to the development of civilizations.

All development is related to what precedes it. Each person has their own developmental history within the larger shared pattern of human motor development. Our personal history of movement patterns and preferences lays the groundwork for how we organize ourselves throughout our life. While developmental movement patterns can be seen as a linear progression, they in fact overlap and interweave as we move from one body organization to another. Patterns appear within patterns and repeat at every stage of development.

Fundamental to the developmental progression is an underlying phenomenon: Patterns of pushing and reaching actions. This pattern-within-pattern of pushing to reaching is reiterated at multiple levels and is basic to our experience. In both our upper and lower bodies, we push before we reach. The push pattern progresses from upper body to lower body and the subsequent reach patterns too, which also progress from the upper body to the lower body. Because our experience of these patterns is so basic to the nature of being human, we even describe people from this fundamental aspect of movement. We talk about someone as being a push over. We may say that a person's reach exceeds his grasp. We are told to boldly reach for the stars. This is yet another example of how our basic biological experience becomes abstracted into metaphoric ideas pertaining to human motivation and interaction.

Try this: Push against the table at which you are sitting. What happens? You feel a sense of pressure that moves you into a direction in space – away from what you are pushing against. The sense of pressure arises from muscle contraction and joint compression. A push condenses the body and is a powerful action. A push is also the preparation for a reach. A clear example of this is the beautiful sequence of a successful jump shot in basketball. The player pushes into the ground with the lower body, which launches the entire body into the air. This push from the lower body initiates a sequence which continues through the upper body through the arms and hands as they extend and reach towards the hoop to make the shot.

Try this: reach across the table at which you are sitting (no, really reach for something, don't just extend your arm!). Contrary to the push, where your body moved away from the table, notice that your body is now moving toward where you are reaching. The sensation is one of extending and expanding.

The organization of our body is achieved through the developmental patterns. With a push you have access to feel the potential of your personal power. With a reach you extend into space and become aware of your relationship to your surroundings. We connect the physical parts of ourselves to our larger selves and our selves to the world around us. This push to reach movement phrase defines the basic duality theme of Self and Other.

Core/Distal Patterning

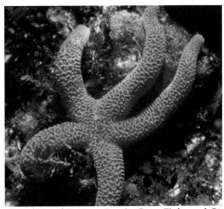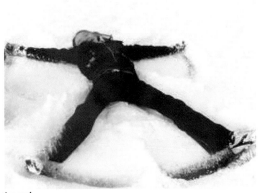

Core/Distal Patterning in Star Fish and Star Angel

A primal pattern of movement connects our central core to the distal ends of our bodies. Like a Sea Anemone whose tentacles contract toward center when stimulated, we organize our spine, arms and legs as though they were actually six limbs: the two spinal limbs of head and tail, as well as two arms and two legs. It is based on our in utero connection between self and mother, in which our center life source is the umbilical cord connection. This pattern establishes the distinction between moving inward toward self and outward toward other. In this pattern, the two ends of the spine and the limbs are equals – they are not differentiated from one another. Try this: the next time you are in bed, condense yourself into a fetal position or a ball shape. Include both ends of your spine so you are as small as possible. Try to feel your six limbs: head, tail, two arms, two legs. Now, from this small ball shape allow the spine to lengthen as you stretch out your arms and legs as wide as possible. This Whole body movement is a necessary precursor for later differentiation of the parts from the Whole, and is still present as an underlying support throughout the developmental progression.

Head/Tail Patterning (Spinal)

Arising from the previous pattern of core/distal connection is a pattern of greater differentiation connecting the two ends of the spine. This is the Head/Tail connection. As vertebrates, our spines form the through line of our length. This is true of all vertebrates, whether the spine is organized in an upright position or in the horizontal position common in most quadrupeds. Whether human, horse or Triceratops, our spines connect our heads to our tails.

When we are born, the spine is in the shape of a "C". It is one continuous curve from head to tail, forming the fetal position. In spinal development and subsequent patterns, the upper body develops before the lower body. As the baby activates his spine, he first learns to support his head, which results in the development of the forward cervical curve. Later, through activation of the lower spine, the baby moves to a sitting position. As the baby learns to support his weight on his lower body, the forward lumbar curve develops. The shape of our spine changes from a single "C" curve to a sequence of balancing curves as a direct result of movement progression.

The spinal pattern connects the large boney containers of the skull, the rib cage and the pelvis and underlies the later, more specific, differentiation between the upper and lower body. Also, because the spine bisects the core of the body, it forms our midline, establishing the right and left sides.

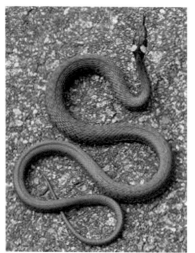 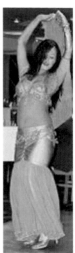

Head/Tail Patterning in snake and belly dancer

The Head/Tail connection is vital to the success of our upright form. Our upright stance, in which we are supported on our two lower limbs, frees our upper bodies to interact with and manipulate the environment. The lower body serves primarily to support and transport us. Think about how you move through your life; your lower body supports your upper body as you move through the world. The lower body takes us from one place to another and supports the upper body in its roles as we sit and think or work and interact. In Rodin's famous sculpture The Thinker, the action of thinking is evident in the pose. The Thinker's head rests in his hand and his arm is supported by his knee in a stable seated position.

However, this role differentiation between the upper and lower body has, in much of contemporary culture, resulted in less reliance on our lower body for locomotion. Most of us in the developed world, no longer use our lower body as our primary mode of transportation, we use our cars and other modes of transport. We don't take the stairs but instead use escalators and elevators. Less reliance on our lower bodies for basic locomotion has resulted in diminished capacity, which in turn can contribute to lower back pain, knee pain, foot issues, etc. It also results in less mobility generally. If we opt out of taking the stairs, taking the stairs becomes increasingly more difficult.

In addition, we are also no longer using our upper body for survival needs such as the hunting and gathering activities of our past. Today upper body actions are often more limited to activities such as checking our Blackberries and punching keypads. Most of us don't do a wide range of physical labor. Less reliance on our upper bodies in fulfilling the primary function of their design also results in diminished capacity, giving rise to a host of upper body maladies including: Temporal-Mandibular Joint (TMJ or jaw) pain, stiff necks and frozen shoulders.

It's not simply that we underutilize our upper body, we frequently overuse small isolated parts, such as when we spend hours typing on keyboards while fixated on a small screen. Isolated, repetitive actions result in overuse syndromes such as eyestrain and Carpal Tunnel Syndrome. We lose the integrity of the Whole of the upper body, which is designed to move in synchrony and in relationship to the core and spine.

The spinal, or Head/Tail, connection between our upper and lower body is part of our expressive design as well as our functional design. When the two ends of the spine fold closer to each other in reflection of our original "C" curve, we are expressing something different than when the spine extends into its vertical length. Our connection to our spine resonates with our sense of self. What do we mean when we say someone is spineless? When we talk about standing up to someone we are referring to the power of the fully developed spine. Try this: drop your head forward while you tuck your tail under. What does this posture remind you of? Now extend both ends of your spine until you are vertical. When do you use this posture? Now what happens if you stick your chest out? Who does this and what does this posture express? Sticking out the chest involves changing the position of the Thoracic or mid section of the spine relative to the two ends.

Upper/Lower Patterning (Homologous)

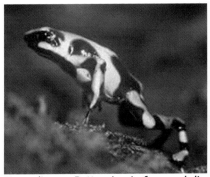 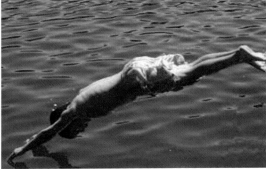

Upper/Lower Patterning in frog and diver

The next step in the developmental progression is the differentiation of the unit of our upper limbs and spine from the unit of our lower limbs and spine. This is the homologous pattern. A good example of the homologous pattern (cited above under **Principles of Development**) can be seen in the action of a basketball player making a jump shot. The player jumps by pushing from his lower body followed by his upper body reaching to make the basket. It can also clearly be seen in the technique of those who skillfully climb coconut palm trees. Their lower body both supports and pushes them upward as their upper body reaches for a higher level. Many basic actions, such as lifting a large box from the floor, and children playing leapfrog, are supported through this pattern. Maximizing the potential for power and strength in homologous movement can also be seen in basic conditioning exercises such as weight lifting, pull-ups and squats. The patterns we see in human development are reiterated in patterns of nature. The actions of rabbits, kangaroos and squirrels are typical examples of this homologous pattern.

Right/Left Patterning (Homolateral)

Another characteristic of our design is our bilateral symmetry. The next developmental pattern differentiates our right and left limbs and right and left sides of the body. Much of how we perceive the world is reflected in this aspect of our design. The two-part pattern of right and left is an essential part of our Wholeness, and of how we perceive and organize our world. It is in the integration of our two sides that we are best able to achieve Wholeness.

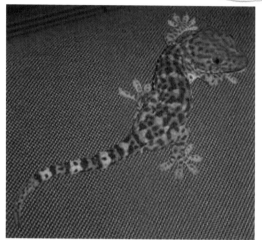 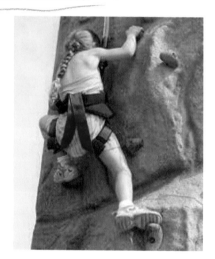

Right/Left Patterning in Gecko and Climber

The two sides reflect both a similarity and difference. While our right and left sides are similar, there is a difference in function and expression of the two sides due to the way our brains work. A right-handed person is both similar to, yet different from, a left-handed person. The right/left contrast is reiterated from the physical body to the abstraction of two sides of an issue. Like the swinging of a pendulum, the rhythm of integrating right and left sides is an ongoing process of both change and continuity.

Having a right and left side contributes to our sense of balance. Imbalance occurs because we overemphasize one side over the other. At the gym, you wouldn't just lift weights with one side of the body! The Scales of Justice suggest that balance is a static place. In reality, balance is in constant flux and requires our constant attention to maintain. If either the right or left side is overly emphasized, imbalance results.

We see every day examples of the homolateral pattern quite frequently when people are in the process of learning new movement skills. This pattern emerges as a preparation for the next, more complex pattern of movement. It can be seen as a reflection of the principle of development that earlier patterns support later patterns and build upon each other.

The homolateral pattern can easily be seen in specialized movement skills such as a cartwheel in gymnastics or sequences of fancy turns in dancing or ice skating. A caricature of this pattern can be seen in the exaggerated swagger of a cowboy, or the lurching walk of Frankenstein's monster. While not always obvious in everyday functional movement, this pattern is a vital underpinning for the more complex contralateral pattern that follows. We must first be able to co-ordinate each side of our body before we can then integrate the two sides. Our experience of our physical duality of having a right side and a left side enables us to understand the nature of duality. We experience the balancing of opposites as a place of peace and well-being; balance takes us back to Wholeness. Try this: first walk with the same arm and leg moving forward at the same time (like the monster of Frankenstein). Now walk normally in your oppositional pattern and really let your arms swing. Note the difference between the homolateral pattern and the final developmental pattern to emerge. . . .

Cross-Lateral Patterning (Contralateral)

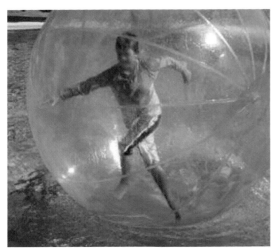 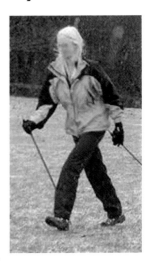

Oppositional Upper/Lower Patterning in running and walking

The contralateral pattern characterizes the human walk, where the opposite arm and leg swing forward with each step. It is the legacy of our arboreal ancestors as they swung from branch to branch. Within this pattern, all the preceding patterns of development are embedded. Earlier patterns clarify subsequent patterns and are always related to each other. Contralaterality is the fulfillment of the human form in that it is the connection of all parts to the Whole: core to distal to head to tail to upper to lower to right to left.

One of the things that characterizes this pattern is the crossing of the mid-line of the body. This movement is significant because it requires the integration of the right and left sides of the body as well as integration of the upper and lower body. It is the pattern that we are designed to use for locomotion. Because we are designed to move forward in space, the contralateral pattern also supports our experience of the depth of front/back. The contralateral pattern is the expression of our ability to access the three dimensions of space.

Repatterning Movement

As stated earlier, movement starts from motivation – whether conscious or not. The initial motivation to move may eventually result in movement patterns that, with many repetitions, become habits. Individual circumstances, personality and experience dictate our movement response and result in our personal movement habits. We don't all brush our teeth exactly the same way, and we don't think about it as we do it. We no longer recall the thinking and physical practice that was required to manipulate the brush to clean our teeth when we were first learning the skill. The learning mode integrates our thinking and sensing selves. Once movement is learned, we are free to think about other things and we lose consciousness of the sensation of moving. We are generally unaware of habitual movement patterns. While sometimes this is beneficial (remember our sock example in Chapter 1) some patterns may one day interfere with our ability to move freely and easily. Our inefficient patterns can be changed, or "repatterned", first by becoming aware of them and then, through exploring alternative movement possibilities for positive change.

Our habitual patterns reflect who we are. The way we stand, the rhythm of our walk, the phrasing and accenting of our speech, our frequent ways of gesturing, all of these (and more) create a portrait of who we are. We have, in essence, a movement signature that characterizes us as members of a specific culture as well as unique individuals.

Look at people around you – some people have feet that are turned out, some have heads that are forward of their shoulders, some have noticeably sway backs, one arm may swing more than the other. We describe people as being "bear-like" or "bird-like", "cat-like" or "rabbit-like". These descriptions reveal aspects of both physical characteristics and personality.

Many things that we associate with "personality" are revealed in a person's individual movement signature. Caricatures such as the stern schoolmarm with set mouth and narrow body posture, or the cowboy with firm bow-legged gait reveal, through movement, what they do and who they are. As do we all. People recognize us not just by how we look, but by how we walk, stand, gesture and interact with others.

Although we generally all have access to a full range of movement, we clearly prefer some ways of moving over others and this is seen in what we do and reflects who we are. Our personal movement signature arises not only from our genes, but also from patterns of our habitual skeletal alignment and our individual movement histories. Are you an athlete, an artist, a scientist? Do you spend more time on your feet or sitting in a chair? What tools do you use: a keyboard, a violin or a lathe? What do you do to relax; read a book or play a round of tennis? Would you rather take a hike through the mountains or lie on a beach? Can you identify yourself as more of a pusher or more of a reacher? All of our activities, whether spontaneous or learned, "inform" our individual forms. While movement patterns can become habits, we can choose to change and repattern our movement once we recognize that we have alternatives.

To summarize, in analyzing the moving body, we can look at parts, such as the skeletal structure and the patterns of human development. However, remember these are just parts of the greater Whole that is human movement and should be considered with respect to how these parts form relationships, patterns and interactions within the Whole.

As we achieve greater mastery over our physical form, we are then able to transcend, therefore abstract our awareness away from the reality of the body. It is this two-edged sword that holds promise for further development as well as the hazard of losing touch with ourselves (our bodies).

The stages of human motor development (much like the geologic layers of the earth) hold our movement history and are the foundation for our present motor patterns. An individual's unique development may have underutilized some early pattern. This deficit will inhibit a more complex later pattern. Therefore, understanding developmental progression allows someone to revisit and repattern specific movements to address deficits and strengths. It is essential to understand the importance of the patterns that serve us, because these patterns organize and support how we connect the parts of ourselves: our upper to lower bodies, our right side to left side and our core to our limbs. These patterns are the blueprint for connecting our parts to our Whole being.

Patterns of the Whole are relationships among the parts. Both differentiation and synthesis are necessary to establish EveryBodies' Wholeness.

Chapter 7

Rotation, Rotation, Rotation

The Beauty of Rotation

Spinal Rotation

Proximal Joint Rotation

Inward and Outward Rotation

The Harmony of Rotation

Chapter 7

Rotation, Rotation, Rotation

"Come on let's twist again like we did last summer, twist again like we did last year"
Chubby Checker

Every good real estate agent knows the value of "location, location, location"! In movement, our slogan is, "rotation, rotation, rotation". Rotation is vital to our survival, as it allows us to scan the full view of our environment. While we do not have the ability to twist our heads like owls, we are able, through our body's rotational abilities, to scan our environment 360 degrees. Whole body rotation is what allows a ballerina to pirouette, the devotional practice of a whirling dervish and the winning degree of difficulty in a gymnast's routine. Rotation enables us to wrap ourselves, or parts of ourselves, around tools and one another. It is the cornerstone of our ability to move three dimensionally in order to fully inhabit our three dimensional world.

The Beauty of Rotation

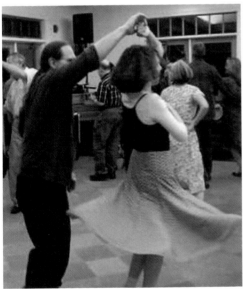

There is something inherently beautiful about rotation. Spinning, twirling, spiraling, twisting, turning - Ferris Wheels, the Wheel of Fortune – the mind-boggling invention of the Wheel! Rotation gives us access to the entire world around us. Rotation allows us to change perspective and provides possibilities. The earth rotates on its axis, and in its orbit, revolves around the sun. Children love to spin, turning round and round until they are dizzy. Rotation creates a circular pathway and the circle is an eternal form; it has no end. A circle is harmonious. A circle creates a safe haven. A circle is a stabilizing container, creating a harmonious balance between Inner and Outer. In a circle, all points are equal, like Knights of the Round Table. The center of a circle could be the center of attention. We circle our wagons, or get lost running in circles. The three dimensional circle becomes the sphere, the coil, the vortex. A spiral or a twist can change everything, or bring us round again. A twister can bring chaos and destruction. The spiral of the double helix holds the code to the human genome.

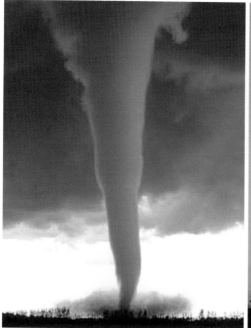 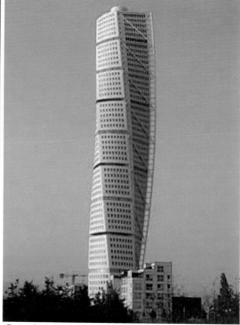

Rotation in nature *Rotation in architecture*

Spinal Rotation

It bears repeating that our spines, as our central vertical core, define our uprightness and our left/rightness. Our access to the spine's ability to rotate is at the heart of our mobility.

The first rotation of a baby's spine, taking him from belly to back or back to belly, signals the end of the mother's peace of mind. At this point, the baby is now mobile and, unless monitored carefully, can roll into trouble! At the other end of life, a diminished capacity for spinal rotation can lead to immobility. This is often the case in older drivers whose ability to rotate decreases, making them unable to safely scan the environment behind them.

Individual parts of the spine, as well as the spine as a Whole, rotate. Earlier, in Chapter 5, we identified sections of the spine's architecture. These sections are different not only in terms of their form, but also in terms of their function. The Cervical Spine has the greatest range of rotation due to the shape and design of the vertebrae that form the curve of the neck. At the top of the cervical spine, at the joint between C1 and C2, we have a pure example of a pivot joint, which allows us to rotate our heads 90 degrees to each side, enabling 180 degrees of total head rotation. The anatomical design of our head/neck and visual system allows us the synergistic capacity to scan our total environment. Most of our sensory organs (eyes, ears, nose, mouth) are situated in the head, so rotation of the head gives us access to the environment and enables us to adapt to our surroundings. This characteristic is reflected in everyday language. Metaphorically, we talk about someone being a real head turner when his attractiveness draws our attention.

Although the rotational capacity of each section of the spine diminishes as we travel down the spine towards the distal end of the Coccyx, the spine as a Whole (along with the Pelvis) has a large range of rotation. Each portion of the spine has a specific design and movement potential, which allows for both subtle and complex movements, optimizing the adaptive capacity of the spine as a Whole.

Proximal Joint Rotation

In addition to our upright stance, we are also defined by our bilateral symmetry. We have two right limbs and two left limbs. Our limbs are connected to our body's core at their proximal joints. The word "proximal" is an anatomical term designating the closest attachment of a limb to the core of the body. Our arms connect to the core through the shoulder girdle and our legs connect to the core through the pelvic girdle. A "distal" joint is one farther away from the core. Our fingers and toes are at the distal ends of our limbs. Elbows and knees are our "mid-limb" joints. The proximal joints of our limbs are ball and socket joints. This type of joint structure allows for the most mobility, both in range and action. Our hip joints, where the ball of the femur (upper leg bone) meets the socket of the pelvis, and our shoulder joints, where the upper arm bone meets the shoulder blade (scapula), provide us with the largest range of motion of any other joints in the body. However, as stated previously, the range of motion in the arms is significantly greater than in the legs due to the structural design of our upper and lower bodies.

One of the reasons physical mobility becomes diminished as we age is because we diminish our movement. For example, because our weight rests on the pelvis when we sit, we lose awareness of the capacity of the pelvis to rotate right and left. The next time you are driving a car, note when you look behind you if you are only rotating your head on the Cervical Spine, or if you are taking advantage of your capacity for rotating the pelvis to get a better view. The capacity for rotation at the spine, the hip and the shoulder joints grants us the ability to move fluidly, gracefully and successfully through our world. Embracing the full rotary action we are endowed with liberates our movement potential.

Inward and Outward Rotation

We have a different experience when twisting or spiraling inward toward our center versus twisting or spiraling outward and away. We twist ourselves into knots, warn someone not to get their "knickers in a twist" or refer to someone's personality as being a little twisted, or abnormal. On the other hand, we also talk about the benefit of "putting a new twist" on something or turning something around to find a solution. We use rotation to connect to ourselves, as well as to connect ourselves to the outside world.

One of the primary ways the parts of our body connect to and relate to each other is through the action of rotation. Like all (apparently) oppositional dualities, inward and outward rotations are two parts of the Whole of rotation. With respect to the limbs, outward rotation is away from our center. Inward rotation is toward our center. Try this: with your arms hanging by your sides in a standing position, rotate your Whole arm outward. This process initially moves the palm forward.

Continue this rotation as far as you can. Be sure to rotate the arm as a Whole, including the shoulder joint, not just the lower arm. Now try to reverse the rotation of the Whole arm inwardly as far as you are able. Inward and outward rotation can give us access to a full 360 degrees of rotation of the Whole arm.

It is possible to achieve even greater mobility of the limbs through the synergistic action of the bony girdles to which they connect. Inward and outward rotation of the arm at the shoulder joint is enhanced through the mobility of the scapula and clavicle (collar bone). The coordinated action of the multiple joints of the shoulder girdle increases the range of motion of the arms and hand, allowing for integrated movement between the distal end of the arm (hand and fingers) and the core of the body.

Our pelvic girdle is also designed to move synergistically with our legs. The joints of the pelvic girdle connect our legs to our spine, and our spine to our legs, thus completing kinetic chains between our upper and lower body and our right and left sides.

Although our upper and lower limbs are similar in some respects, remember we do not have the same range of motion in the lower body that we do at the upper. This is because our lower body is designed for greater stability in its role as base of support. Our upper body is designed for greater mobility, enabling us to interact with the world through our use of tools, instruments and gestures.

The Harmony of Rotation

There is a balance and harmony among the rotations of our body parts. For example, our right and left sides frequently rotate in opposition. This is in harmony with our upright stance and bipedal locomotion, which altogether results in our basic walking pattern. From a macro point of view, walking is primarily a flexion and extension pattern. However, walking includes a subtle combination of oppositional rotation of the proximal joints and spine. This harmonious rotation is what gives a walk its grace and fluidity.

Try this: walk across the room and let your arms and legs swing freely and easily. Try to emphasize the potential to spiral through the upper body. Now walk carefully and try to eliminate all twisting. Observe that this makes the walk more stiff and robotic.

When we turn our head, whether to say "No" or to check for oncoming traffic, we are actually rotating the upper (cervical) spine. Our heads turn and our rib cage and our pelvis rotate, due to their attachment to the spine. The degree of spinal rotation varies from the head to the pelvis, but the combined synergy of all of our moveable vertebrae rotating right or left allows our Whole body an amazing range of motion.

Try this: Stand with the legs shoulder width apart. Starting from the head, rotate to the right and gradually allow the rotation to sequence down through the shoulders, ribs and finally the Whole pelvis. (The ribs have to rotate because they are connected to the thoracic spine. The pelvis has to rotate because it is connected to the spine at the sacrum. You may recall that the sacrum is composed

68

of fused vertebrae and is both part of the spine and part of the pelvis). Continue to rotate the Whole body by allowing the right leg to rotate outward while the left leg follows along, inwardly rotating. Be sure to allow both legs to rotate fully, letting the feet pivot on the floor. All of these combined rotations within the body will allow you to twist 360 degrees! Were you successful? **The rotations of all these parts allow the rotation of the body as a Whole, in the same way that individual instruments produce the harmony of a symphony.**

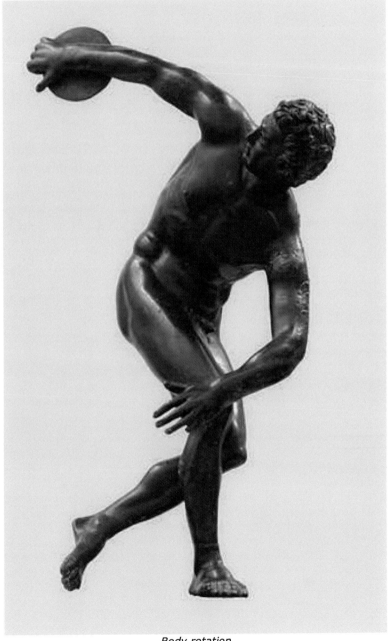

Body rotation

The anatomical action of rotation also works synergistically with the other body actions of flexion, extension, abduction and adduction in creating Whole body integrated movement. Try this: start from a standing position, arms hanging by your sides. Rotate the right arm outward, away from the body, as the left arm rotates inward, toward the body. Keep this action going until the Whole body begins to spiral. You will undoubtedly notice that the tendency is for the body to turn toward the direction of the right outwardly rotating arm. Now try this: allow both arms to rotate inwardly toward the body. Keep the action going and allow the upper spine, including the head, to respond to this action. You will probably note that the head and spine have rounded and dropped forward. Now, if you reverse the action of rotation, turning the arms outward away from the body, note how the spine responds by extending, resulting in an arching action up and back.

The Whole body integration of the above movement sequences illustrates the patterns of kinetic chains of action. Although we can move body parts in isolation, the functional efficiency of Whole body movement is supported through the synergy of kinetic chain action. Rotation is a crucial element in these patterns and is built into the design of human movement.

The ability of our bodies to rotate as we move from cradle to grave keeps us healthy and mobile. It is among the most effective and simple movement "prescriptions" we can give for retaining and regaining optimal function. Re-learn and re-visit the patterns of childhood by twisting, turning, spinning and rolling. Whenever you are feeling stuck, rotate. Throughout the day, find moments to rotate your wrists and hands. Do slow small circles from the top of the head. Stand up and do your own version of the "60's" Twist. (Why do you suppose The Twist was such a huge hit?) Circle your feet. Roll your shoulders. Find ways to incorporate more rotation into your life. Understanding, appreciating and experiencing the body's full capacity for rotation is vital for a continuing good quality of life as we age.

Remember this simple mantra: When in doubt, rotate! Rotation helps us to adapt, provides alternatives and helps us to see a bigger picture. Furthermore, rotation helps EveryBody maintain mobility over the course of their entire lives.

Chapter 8

Our Core in Relation to the Whole

Defining Core

The Principle of Core Support

Some Physical Facts of Core Support

Pelvic Core

Chapter 8

Our Core In Relation To The Whole

"The good man is he who exemplifies in his movement physical, mental, emotional and spiritual values as a unified whole." Rudolf Laban

Defining Core

True understanding requires getting to the heart of the matter. The heart, the roots, the core, the center, are terms we use metaphorically to signify the fundamental essence of something. From atoms to apples to art, core is synonymous with what is most vital to the Whole. The human body can lose limbs and still live, but profound damage to vital organs is fatal. As a survival mechanism, the body shuts down at the periphery in order to save what is core. This is why frostbite begins at the fingers and toes.

What is core? Things which come to mind include: The core of an apple, the core of the earth, core values, core ingredients. Core is something that is at the center and essential to the Whole. A general association is that the body's core is the abdominal musculature. Anyone who goes to a gym or reads fitness articles has been made aware of the emphasis on developing a "strong core". The

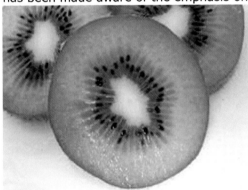

popularity of Pilates-based workouts also exemplifies this trend in the fitness industry. But there is more at the center of the body and essential to the Whole than simply skeletal muscle. For example, the front (anterior) of the spine is located at the center of the body. The Thoracic Diaphragm, our principle muscle of breathing, is centrally located. The digestive organs are at the core of the body (think of the impact a full meal has on your desire to move!).

Is the heart part of our core? Is the brain in some way core? And then there are more poetic aspects of the body's core. To have a gut reaction and to be broken-hearted are examples of our emotional and intuitive center. What is vital to us physically, intellectually, emotionally, and spiritually is at our core and defines us as unique individuals. Things that we consider to be core are related to aspects of self and in some sense, core is self. Core is deep, core is profound. The Earth contains an active and mobile core within its many layers. The core of a fruit holds the seed for the next harvest. It is in the central issues of a dispute that resolution can be found. All of these images share a common bond.

Above we have used the terms "core" and "center" interchangeably. But are they? Is core the same as center? Yes and no. The idea of center implies a logical, theoretical, mathematical notion of relative location. The center of gravity is the point where weight is concentrated in a body or structure; the center of a circle is a point equidistant from all points on the circumference of the circle; one's spiritual center is a metaphor for the meaningfulness around which belief systems are organized. Center then, is often an abstraction, an idea – a mental construct. Core, on the other hand, exists physiologically. The core of the body is what is essential to survival. Mountain climbers may lose fingers and toes in conditions of extreme cold because the body shuts off what is expendable or non-essential to fundamental life processes.

The developmental process we discussed in Chapter 6 moves from core to periphery and from simple to complex. As we develop into increasing complexity, our parts become more specialized and differentiated. The upside of this is the evolution of potential. The downside of this is that we lose our sense of Wholeness. Our complexity provides us with a lot of opportunity, but the flip side is, in isolating a part we often mistake it for the Whole. This often results in a loss of connection or relationship to what is essential – our core. Loss of connection to our core may arise from many sources, including (but not limited to) the psychological, cultural, experiential, and personal parts of the Whole of one's life.

Our physical, sensory experience of our core, leads to our understanding of core as located at the center of the body. However, it is not only a location. It is the beginning from which we develop. It is the foundation from which all life is generated. Core is the nucleus of the single cell, from which all development unfolds. The perspective of core as biologically based distinguishes linguistically the notions of "core" from "center". When discussing aspects of core, we need to be clear about what core is the "core of." Core describes a relationship of parts to Whole; therefore we need to understand the context.

For example, in a fitness regime that advocates core strengthening – what is being strengthened in relationship to what and for what purpose? Strong abdominal muscles are just a part of the picture. Core as a relationship brings into focus all of the physiological aspects of connection that together form true core support. Frequently, lower back pain is not simply a matter of weak abdominal muscles. Strengthening muscle may play a part in reducing pain, but without taking into account the **WholeMovement** patterning of the individual, the problem will not be fully addressed. The stabilizing and mobilizing of the body's core in relationship to its periphery, the dynamic phrasing of movement, and the alignment of parts throughout a movement process, are just some aspects that may actually be the source of chronic pain.

The Principle of Core Support

So what then, is core support in terms of movement? The Principle of Core Support involves bringing what is vital to movement into relationship. Our core skeletal structure of head, rib cage and pelvis comes into relationship through the spine. The many vertebrae of our spine in the center of our body come into relationship through connection of the head and tail (coccyx). Our organs fill the container of our torso and contribute to our sensation of movement. We move due to the relationship between muscular strength and flexibility. We stand up and locomote through the balancing of our center of gravity over our base of support. There are many, many models of looking at how the parts of the body organize into Wholeness.

Different ideas of physiological core arise from these different perspectives. Each perspective has something to offer, but is incomplete in and of itself. For example, think about how you differentiate your lower body from your upper body. Where does your "upper" body end and your "lower" body begin? How and where do they meet or merge? Perhaps you think of your waist as the dividing line between upper and lower. Is this because your waist is at the level of your navel? Or is it because your waist is above your hips and below your ribs? There is some truth to the idea that waist is core, but it is not the Whole truth. Keep in mind that the "waist" is not actually an anatomical structure! In the notion of waist as core, we are conflating the experience of the middle of the body with what is core to the moving body. In another example, go back to the idea that the Thoracic Diaphragm (our principle breathing muscle) is the location of the core because it forms the ceiling of the abdomen and the floor of the thorax. This is also partially true, but since the Thoracic Diaphragm moves up and down, the location of core is always changing relative to the Whole as we breathe. Fitness professionals often cite specific muscles like the Transverse Abdominus and the Iliopsoas as core. While these muscles are important, they are only part of the complex pattern of muscular interaction, in kinetic chains, that contributes to core support of the body.

Some Physical Facts of Core Support

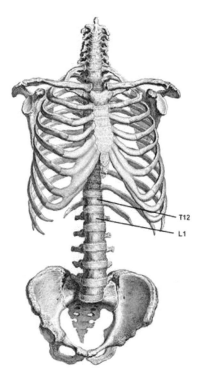

Pelvis in relationship to spine

So, if the above examples give only part of the picture, what is the Whole of the concept of core? Using the metaphor of the creamy center of an Oreo cookie, our body's core is both the filling and the connection between the two chocolate cookies. The center of our body is composed of bone, muscle, organs and other tissues. While these structures can be differentiated for purposes of analysis, they functionally interact in myriad, overlapping, interweaving patterns.

Starting from our skeletal structure, there is a vital significance to the meeting place between the last Thoracic Vertebra (T12) and the first Lumbar Vertebra (L1). It is here that the backward thoracic curve starts to change to the forward lumbar curve and where the mobility of the spine increases. This boney meeting place of T12 to L1 can be considered a skeletal part of our Core Support. This is also the location of crucial connections of the Thoracic Diaphragm and Iliopsoas muscles! (Once again, parts in relationship.)

Looking further at muscular aspects of core, it is revealing to look at the geographical relationships of our deepest muscles. Together they support our three dimensional form moving three dimensionally. These muscles connect our upper and lower parts to our right and left parts to our front and back parts. In addition to the Thoracic Diaphragm and Iliopsoas; the Transversalis, Quadratus Lumborum and the muscles of the Pelvic Floor weave together, forming both the muscular container and content of the body's core.

When the Thoracic Diaphragm descends during inspiration, pressure is put on the organs of digestion. The ongoing, overlapping rhythms within and among the organs of respiration, digestion and blood flow interact in the ongoing Whole of the movement of life. When you have to wait to empty your bladder, you probably experience the building of pressure as a change in bodily rhythms. Tightened muscles, diminished breath and urgency may be translated into small vibratory actions. During labor and delivery, mothers are coached in using their breath rhythms to aid uterine contractions. We tend to associate our muscles as the engines that move us, but all of our tissues are inter-related. Whenever our parts are not moving optimally, it results in hampering the movement of the body as a Whole. A runner with a stitch in his side, a football player with wind knocked out of him, and anyone experiencing abdominal cramps, feels the truth of the organs as a vital part of core support for movement.

Pelvic Core

What and where, exactly, is the pelvis? The pelvis is a large bowl of bone that contains vital viscera. It is centrally located, the bridge between the upper and lower body. Functionally, it corresponds with our weight center (center of gravity). The pelvis and the spine intersect at a triangular bone called the sacrum. The name of this bone means "sacred". This is appropriate because of its location and function in the body. It forms both the back of the pelvis and the base of the spine. The sacrum is composed of fused vertebrae and is the point at which weight from the spine is transferred through the pelvic bowl downward to the legs.

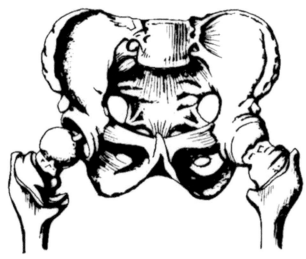

Pelvis in relation to lower limbs

The pelvis both supports and transmits our weight, while also being highly mobile. This dual role of stability and mobility is what gives the pelvis its power. As we said earlier, in the skeleton, mobility occurs at joints. Another name for joint is "articulation". We think of someone as being "articulate" when he or she has a facile command of language. We can think of an articulate mover as someone with a facile command of the movement of their joints. The highly articulate pelvis gets its mobility from the joints that connect it to the legs and spine. The pelvis' connection to the lumbar spine (lower back) and its connection to the ball and socket joints at the top of the legs allow the bowl to really rock and roll. "Elvis the Pelvis" was a master of this!

Try this: Take a moment now to stand up and move your pelvic bowl. Let your knees be slightly bent and place your hands on your hips (the sides of the bowl). It is important for the knees to stay relaxed in order to experience the free movement of the pelvis where it connects to the legs. Imagine that your pelvis is filled with water. Try tipping the bowl in different directions, allowing the water to pour out. Also try keeping the bowl level while twisting from side to side without spilling any water. Repeat the above with your knees straight. Do you feel the difference?

We interfere with pelvic power by fixing it in a rigid habitual postural pattern. Remember that skeletal alignment is dynamic and constantly changing to meet our needs. Remember too, that the pelvis connects our upper and lower bodies so it must be available to both move us and support us. Think back to the Head/Tail Connection discussed in Chapter 6. The Head and Tail maintain connection through the pelvis. For instance, to sit down or stand up, the two ends of the spine counterbalance one another, but the pelvis is what moves our weight through the space. The pelvis, as our center of weight, always moves in relationship to the Whole. A good basketball player knows to watch his opponent's pelvis in order to anticipate what his next move will be. We go wherever our pelvis leads us.

There is no one correct position of the pelvis. Many problems stem from "locking" the pelvis into a fixed position, creating immobility. Examples of this include an exaggerated sway back (the pelvic bowl is tipped forward, creating compression of the lumbar spine) or the reverse, in which the tail is tucked under. Try this: first walk with the pelvis in the position with the tail tucked underneath you. Next walk with an exaggerated sway back with the tail reaching backward. Can you find the neutral middle ground in which the pelvis hangs freely? Does one of these alignments seem more familiar?

Efficient function of the pelvis requires a balance between these extremes. In your daily actions of walking up stairs and getting into your car, take a moment to become aware that the pelvis is propelling you through the space. Playing with a hula-hoop is a great way to become more aware of, and to fully mobilize your pelvis. You also may notice that your Whole self feels better.

The structure and location of the pelvis is core to the body's architecture, and the power of the pelvis is core to human movement. It is core as the center of our weight, which makes it possible to move through space. It is core as the connector of our upper and lower body. It is core as the container of vital organs. It is core as the source of our seed, like the core of an apple. It is core as the origin of our "gut response". Both literally and metaphorically, the pelvis is home to our expressive selves. It simultaneously contains the essence of self and propels that self through space.

However, the core of the human body is not just the structures of bone, muscle and organs. It is rather, the relationship among these structures, as well as our sense of self. When we speak metaphorically about core beliefs and values, we are connecting our physical experience of embodiment to the mental constructs of what it means to be human.

Experiencing the body's core, particularly the structure and function of the pelvis, gives EveryBody access to the vitality of life. Our core is both our stable and mobile center, from which we connect to ourselves and the world around us.

Chapter 9

The Dynamic Expression of Movement

The *How* of Movement

The Dynamic Qualities of Movement

The Quality of Flow as a Dynamic of Movement

The Quality of Force as a Dynamic of Movement

The Quality of Time as a Dynamic of Movement

The Quality of Attending as a Dynamic of Movement

Combining Qualities of Movement Dynamics

Phrasing the Dynamics of Movement

Dynamic Fulfillment

Chapter 9

The Dynamic Expression Of Movement

"The flow of effort from the weightless, timeless, spaceless centre to the matter shaped and moved around is the binding link which carries life." Rudolf Laban

The *How* of Movement

We have talked about "*what*" is moving: our body. The "*how*" of movement is its quality and dynamics - that which gives movement its color and tone. Movement quality sets the mood and underscores the mover's intent. A gentle caress of the face and a slap of the face consist of the same use of body and space. What differs is the energy used, which expresses two very different motivations. The colors, or dynamic palette of our movement, serve us both expressively and functionally. You may start to remove a crumb from the table with a light brushing action, but if it sticks, you will have to use more force to rub it away. While it is easy to name body parts and to map spatial directions (right arm reaching up), the infinite variety and subtleties of the energy of our movement is less quantifiable.

A basic description of movement can be as simple as, "he walked into the room". But this tells us nothing about why or how the person walked into the room. Did he stride purposefully? Did he sneak into the room? Was his walk free and easy, or were his steps careful and restrained? When you hear footsteps, you can often tell something about the mover's intention or mood by the quality of the sound. Is he in a hurry, or taking his time? It is also possible to recognize someone by hearing the approaching footsteps. As the Beatles said, "something in the *way* she moves" can identify a unique individual.

The Dynamic Qualities of Movement

Remember that we define movement as **"patterns of change".** When there is a change in energy, there is movement. What then, are the qualities of movement? The answer lies in how we change the ways in which we organize and expend energy. This includes how we focus our attention in the world around us; how we express the passage of time; how we exert control; and how much force we use. Changes in the use of, and type of, energy contribute to the range of movement possibilities. For instance, there are some actors who are known for the wide range of characters they are able to portray. There are other actors who always seem to play the same type of role. The difference between them is the dynamic range they bring to creating a character. Sylvester Stallone has achieved fame and fortune by playing a very particular and narrow range of character qualities. Meryl Streep is known for her ability to portray a wide range of characters. While we are all capable of a range of expressive choices, our personal movement signature reveals our "color" preferences and habits. Just as singers have different vocal ranges and styles, we as movers have varying ranges of dynamic expression.

Personality "types" are frequently descriptions of a distinctive way in which energy is used and changed. What words would you use to describe the cheerleader, the jock and the nerd? The cheerleader might be described as bubbly, bouncy, out-going and energetic. She might also be described as superficial, air-headed and snobby. The jock might be described as a wholesome all-American good guy, or a bully. The nerd might describe himself as intelligent, logical, and sensitive; while to others he might seem to be awkward, a pushover and painfully shy. In each case, we have described two opposing characterizations of a type. These oppositions might be considered positive vs. negative descriptions. It is interesting that the same movement characteristics can evoke polar opposite views of a personality type. It is not the movement, but rather our interpretation of the movement, that gives rise to meaning. This is just one reason why treatises on "body language" can be misleading. The meaning of movement depends on a constantly changing set of contexts, in tandem with the perception of the observer.

The point is, our perception and experience determine how we interpret the dynamics of movement in others. The more quantifiable aspects of movement having to do with Body and Space are comparable to prose. But descriptions of the qualitative dynamics of movement are the poetry of motion. In our example above, one can make the statement, "he walked into the room". But how much more meaningful and interesting it is to say, "he swaggered belligerently", "strode purposefully", "limped painfully", or "crept stealthily into the room". Body and Space tell you what and where, but the energy used conveys how and even why.

The Quality of Flow as a Dynamic of Movement – Holding On or Letting Go

In Chapter 1 we discussed flow from the larger perspective of the flow of life itself. While flow can be considered from this macro point of view, it can also be examined from a more micro perspective with respect to how we modulate our personal flow. Flow is the baseline of ongoing energy that changes to meet our functional and expressive needs. Flow is how we control the progression of movement. In certain instances, a great deal of control is necessary for success: putting a contact lens into your eye, carrying a tray of full drink glasses across a room, threading a needle. In other instances, the success of the action lies in flow's unrestrained outpouring: waving to get someone's attention, a big sigh of relief, hurling an object. Throughout our day, our flow is constantly fluctuating on a continuum between release and control, between holding on and letting go. In the vocabulary of Laban Movement Analysis, we differentiate between degrees of Free Flow and Bound Flow.

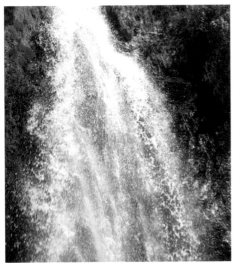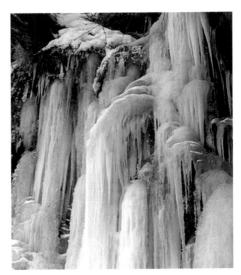

Images suggesting Free and Bound Flow

While flow serves us both functionally and expressively, it should come as no surprise that some people tend more toward the controlling side of flow, and others tend toward a more relaxed use of flow. A person with more controlled flow (Bound Flow) can be seen as either rigid or careful. A person who prefers the opposite side of flow (Free Flow) can be seen as "easy-going" or irresponsible. Once again, perspective and context will determine how appropriate someone's personal use of flow appears, and how it serves her. Also, while one may prefer one side of the flow spectrum to its opposite side, the fact is that we all vary and modulate our use of flow to some degree. Flow is the baseline of our movement. Awareness of flow contributes to the ease and efficiency of movement.

Try this: To feel the difference between Bound and Free Flow, first take a deep breath in and gradually and evenly let the air out. Now repeat, but this time let the air rush out all at once. Under what circumstances would each of these breath patterns serve you functionally? What does each express? Now reach your arm over your head and hold it there. First carefully and gradually return your arm to where it started. Once again extend your arm over your head. This time release your arm, allowing it to simply drop. While gravity actually caused the arm to drop, your intention to release and let go initiated the movement.

The Quality of Force as a Dynamic of Movement – A Firm Grip or a Delicate Touch?

The way in which we exert force is another functional and expressive aspect of our movement. When you slap your friend's hand in a high five gesture, you use a different amount of force than when you brush something off of his face. We are constantly varying how we exert force as we go about our daily tasks, but there is always an expressive component operating as well. Like Flow, the use of force takes place along a continuum, with one extreme being a Strong exertion, increasing pressure, and the other extreme being a Light and delicate decrease of pressure. Try this: using one hand, gently and as lightly as possible, brush your fingers over the skin of your other arm just barely brushing the hairs. Now gradually increase pressure until you are rubbing your arm with strength, really manipulating the deeper tissues. Now gradually decrease this pressure until you are once again delicately touching your arm.

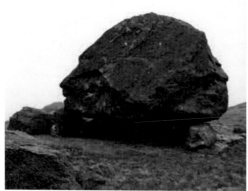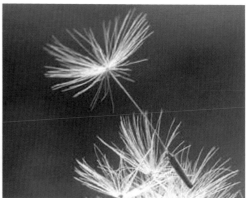

Images suggesting Strong and Light Force

Think about times when you use a delicate touch versus the occasions when you apply yourself forcefully. In order to move a heavy piece of furniture, you first test how much force is necessary to overcome the resistance of the object. We have all had the experience of using more force than is required, sometimes with humorous results! How many times has Charlie Brown fallen flat on his back when Lucy pulls away the football right before he makes contact? It is also surprising when you try to pop a balloon and find that much more force is required than you expected.

The way in which you exert force is a component of personal expression. Some individuals are most at home at the Strong end of the spectrum, while others tend toward the Light end. We have positive or negative attitudes about how and when we exert force. However, both ends of the spectrum can be equally effective and reveal personality styles. Who do you know with a strong personality? This person uses a firm hand, puts his foot down, and can't be budged on an issue. This can be seen as authoritative or authoritarian and, while effective at times, it is only one strategy and may not work at all in other situations. At the other end of the continuum, whom do you know that is a "steel magnolia", a person who applies her will and gets her way with a delicate touch? The art of negotiation may require both increasing and decreasing pressure to get results.

Exertion of force is aligned with personal empowerment. This brings us to confusions that surround the word "weight". Our bodies have weight. In this case the term is a quantitative measurement. We lose weight and we gain weight. However, weight is also a metaphor having qualitative meaning for how we assert ourselves in the world. Something "heavy" is considered more serious, while something "light" is considered less serious. One can have a heavy heart or be light hearted. When you express an opinion, you weigh in on a matter. An aggressive person might be accused of throwing his weight around. A light weight is a push over!

The Quality of Time as a Dynamic of Movement –
Not Enough Time or Plenty of Time

We have all had the experience of waiting for something to happen. Time seems to drag on endlessly. You check your watch again to discover that only five minutes have passed since you last checked! Conversely, all of us have experienced being so totally involved in something that three hours have passed, seemingly in the blink of an eye. In both of these instances, our experience of passing time is distinct from the discreet measurements of time ticking by. We measure time quantitatively in seconds, minutes, weeks, years, and eons. But time can also be considered qualitatively, revealed in the mover's attitude toward the passage of time. Do you know someone who always seems to be rushing? Have you recently felt the frustration of being waited on by a store clerk who dawdles? How we feel about the time we have, whether with an attitude of urgency or an attitude of leisurely lingering, is a quality that colors our movement. Remember that time, as a quality of movement, is not about being fast or slow. Our movement can be fast without our feeling a sense of urgency about accomplishing it. A professional chef may chop vegetables in the blink of an eye while exuding a leisurely attitude. Our movement can be slow without our intending to indulge in the moment. Someone disarming an explosive device will move slowly, but will probably feel a sense of urgency about his actions. Movement is change. As your attitude toward time changes (whether you are conscious of it or not) the quality of your movement changes.

Imagine that a glass is falling off the table. You have a sense of urgency that causes you to accelerate to catch the glass before it hits the floor. Immediately afterwards you may feel a sense of relief that causes your movement to change toward sustainment. Notice that these changes in your attitude toward time are related to a decision – a decision to accelerate followed by a decision to decelerate. This is an example of the often unconscious functional aspect of the quality of time.

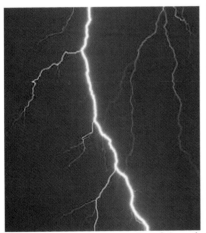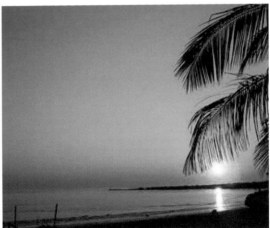

Images suggesting urgent or leisurely attitude toward Time

Someone who frequently expresses an urgent attitude toward time may be either an enthusiastic go-getter or anxious and stressed out. A person whose attitude toward time is one of indulgence may be either calm and serene, or lazy and indolent. How do you personally experience time? When are you eager to "get on with it", and when would you rather linger awhile?

The Quality of Attending as a Dynamic of Movement – Taking it All In or Single Focus

A successful quarterback needs to be aware of the entire playing field, while a pro golfer making a crucial putt needs to be single focused. In one case, the football player has to attend to the Whole of the immediate environment. In the other case, the golfer has to exclude everything in the environment except a specific goal. An effective speaker has the ability to fluctuate between attending to the entire audience and attending to a single individual, which enhances his ability to communicate.

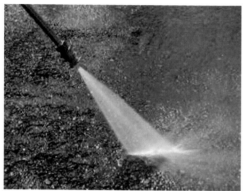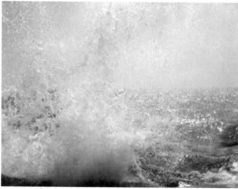

Images suggesting single focus and all-encompassing focus

Attention to the environment, while frequently associated with eye focus, reflects the mover's attitude toward his surroundings rather than simply his use of vision. While our eyesight is our primary sensory mode of attending to the environment, it is only a part of the process of attending. For example, think about trying to navigate through a room in the dark. You have your feelers out in order to avoid bumping into the furniture. When you smell a pleasant smell or hear an unusual sound, these senses also contribute to a change in your awareness of the environment.

Try this: pretend you are sowing grass seed. At first, make sure you sprinkle handfuls of seed in an attempt to completely and evenly spread the seed. Now, mime you are planting a single seed in a specific spot in the soil. You have now changed the quality of your movement from attending to the whole environment to an exclusive specificity. You could accomplish this movement change with your eyes closed. Certain jobs require one to keep track of many things as they occur simultaneously (a receptionist in a busy environment) while other jobs require concentrated single focus (a microbiologist conducting a lab test). Do you know someone who sees the big picture and takes it all in? Do you know someone who is great with details? Perhaps you know someone who is often spaced out, seemingly out of touch with what is going on around him? When and how do you attend to the world around you? As with all the qualities of movement, some qualities are more a part of our personal movement signature and are linked to how we perceive the world.

Combining Qualities of Movement Dynamics

Above we have described four movement Factors, each having two opposite expressions: Bound or Free Flow; Light or Strong application of Force; a Sudden or Sustained attitude toward Time; and a Direct or Flexible attention to the immediate environment. However, movement is very complex and the dynamics of movement are constantly in flux, occurring in combination and changing from moment to moment. For instance, in the example of the pro golfer making the crucial putt, he not only uses Direct Attention toward the goal, he also controls his Flow. The sequence of actions, as the golfer accomplishes his putt, is composed of complex changes in the intensity and combination of movement qualities, as well as changes in his body's organization in space.

Much of everyday movement is not very dynamic. Look around at people in line in a grocery store. You may observe people shifting weight, and perhaps variations in the degree of spatial awareness. But it is not a good example of dynamic movement compared with the drama of a sporting event or a rock concert. In our everyday language, we don't tend to use the full vocabulary available to us. The same is true of our movement choices. We are not always calling upon the full range of dynamic choices available to us. A larger vocabulary enables you to communicate more effectively, both in word choice and movement choice.

In order to move with the greatest range available to you, it is helpful first to be familiar with your dynamic preferences. If you are aware that you are a person who does not prefer attending to the environment, simply reminding yourself that you can open your awareness to "the big picture" around you, can change your outlook, mood and perspective. Becoming aware of the ability to free your flow can assist you in releasing habitual holding patterns that result from stress. As we have said earlier, any change in a part produces a change in the Whole. Habitual patterns of the qualities of movement can be replaced with new patterns that are more effective. This may lead to better health and a greater sense of well being.

Phrasing the Dynamics of Movement

You may recall in Chapter 1, one of the primary patterns was phrasing. In the phrasing of our movement, what we emphasize, or accentuate through dynamic qualities, contributes to its meaning. Try this: Say the following sentence, "I believe this is yours". Where did you place the emphasis? Now try emphasizing the bold word below:

I believe this is yours.
I believe **this** is yours.
I believe this is **yours**.

Where and how emphasis occurs in a phrase changes the meaning in our actions as well as in our words. Emphasis supports meaning and can be created in a number of ways. Emphasis can occur through duration. For instance, when you emphasized the first word in the sentence above, did you linger and draw out the word "I", or did you make it abrupt and forceful? Emphasis can also be created through loading. Loading means adding more layers of expression. For example, the dynamics of a movement can be Direct and Quick (like an action used to pop a bubble), or an action could be more loaded, with the addition of Strong force, as in a Punch (Direct, Quick and Strong). A caress could be delicate and Free, but adding Sustained time will load the moment by drawing it out (Light, Free, Sustained).

Another way emphasis within a phrase occurs is through accenting. Accenting connects to the rhythm of a phrase, giving it a distinct pattern. Try this: tap a little repetitive rhythm with your hand. Can you identify the accents? Duration and loading contribute to the accents and rhythm of our movement. Where emphasis occurs contributes to the expressiveness of the phrase. Repeat the three spoken phrases above. Did you feel how the meaning changed, depending on where and how the emphasis was placed?

Emphasis placed at the beginning of a phrase can have an explosive or impulsive feel. An Impulsive Phrase can drive you into action, but it may also be an impulse that puts you in jeopardy. A leap of faith refers to the positive aspect of an Impulsive Phrase. Look before you leap is an admonition warning of the consequences of an impulsive action.

Emphasis at the end of a phrase is impactive. A heated argument may end with a big blowup, such as the slamming of a door, or a punch. An Impactive Phrase is a building to a climax. A climax can be achieved by any change in dynamics that emphasizes the end of a phrase. It is the exclamation point at the end of the sentence, the cymbal crash. It can also be a powerful or poignant ending, as in a moment of revelation, inspiring awe.

Emphasis in the middle of a phrase creates a swing. Like waves on the shoreline that approach, break, and then recede, a Swing Phrase is loaded or accented in the middle. Children like to swing because the suspended moment in the middle is a pleasurable anticipation of the downward rush. A swing can also be an endless recycling without moving onward.

A phrase with no emphasis is even. An even phrase is not without meaning. Perhaps you have been bored or frustrated by a teacher who drones on using only long, Even Phrasing. However, a measured even tone can be useful to calm a frightened child or restore order to a potentially volatile situation.

We are capable of all types of dynamic phrasing. However, like most movement patterns, we all have preferences that are part of our personal movement signature. What type of phrasing feels most comfortable for you? When you repeated the sentence above, was there one type of phrasing that felt more natural to you? The dynamics of our phrasing can be seen not only in our moment-to-moment actions, but also in the larger patterns of our lives. Is your day loaded at the beginning, the middle or the end? Do you bounce out of bed in the morning, or are you more of a night person? Who do you know that you would describe as impulsive or impactive?

In movement, phrases are accented, or loaded, through changes in the dynamic qualities we discussed above. An Impulsive Phrase is more dynamic at the beginning. A Swing Phrase is more dynamic in the middle. An Impactive Phrase is more dynamic at the end. In an Even Phrase, there is no dynamic change.

Think about people you know who you would describe as dynamic, "larger then life" or charismatic. Can you identify some of the dynamic qualities we have discussed? A dynamic speaker or performer draws us in because of their ability to modulate and vary their dynamic range.

Dynamic Fulfillment

Humans crave dynamic expression and seek pleasure through dynamic variation. We add spice to our foods. We invest in the color, texture and pattern of fabrics. How we dress, how we decorate, and what we choose to do reflects dynamic choice which expresses personal style. Although we need and seek dynamic variation, contemporary society frequently encourages limited dynamics of movement. From an early age we are taught to keep quiet and sit still. In addition, the routines of many jobs don't require dynamic variation, and are actually more efficient without much dynamic variation, whether working on a computer or an assembly line. As life becomes increasingly complex, we fragment parts of the Whole into more and more specializations, thus losing our ability to access the full range of our movement dynamics.

We are drawn to artistic expression because, in part, it fulfills the human craving for dynamic range. One attends the symphony in order to experience the dynamic qualities of the music. The dynamics of the music are achieved through the dynamic range of movement of both the musicians and the conductor. Likewise, we go to a sporting event to see the physical exuberance and dynamic range of the athletes. Most entertainment relies on the desire of the observer to experience a full dynamic range of movement. That's one reason why we pay for tickets to scary movies and raucous comedies.

While it is wonderful that we have access to the pleasures derived from the expertise of artists, athletes and designers, there is a danger that we become consumers and observers rather than participants in the dynamics of life. This becomes increasingly true as virtual experience replaces actual experience.

Our appreciation of the highly skilled abilities that specialization gives us is a good thing. However, we suggest that you can have your cake and eat it too. In fact, your appreciation of these highly skilled abilities can be enhanced through your own experience with the dynamic range of movement. Freedom to express yourself is necessary to your well-being. Finding opportunities for this is an essential (and often challenging) part of modern life.

Dynamics is the cornerstone of expression. Expression is the cornerstone of communication. Having access to the full range of our body's expressive movement assists EveryBody in communicating and interacting.

Chapter 10

The Body's Shape - Container and Content

Familiar Shape Forms

The Shape of Body Attitude

Moving our Shape – The Mode of Shape Flow

Moving our Shape – The Mode of Bridging to the Environment

Moving our Shape – The Mode of Molding and Adapting

Shape Qualities – Change in the Core

Affinities and Disaffinities between Shape and Space

Shape as Both Container and Content

Chapter 10

The Body's Shape – Container and Content

"In the long run, we shape our lives, and we shape ourselves. The process never ends until we die." Eleanor Roosevelt

We are always moving, so the body's shape is always changing. However, we tend to associate the idea of shape as something that is fixed or stable, unmoving. In actuality we are always changing and accommodating to the present moment, yet the next moment is always emerging.

A shape that has intrigued artists and scientists for centuries is the Mobius strip. It is a shape that beautifully represents something we intuitively understand; the paradox of duality. When you run your finger along the form of the Mobius strip, one side becomes the other side as the inner surface becomes the outer surface. You can make a Mobius strip by simply taking a narrow strip of paper, twisting it once and taping the ends together.

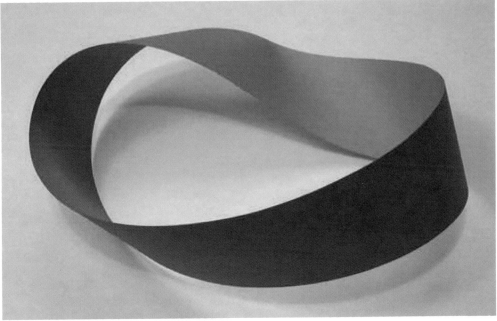

Mobius strip

While our shape is always changing, the notion of static forms is a way we perceive and assign meaning to our world. We recognize the shape of a cat, a tree, a house, a rock, a car, in part through our perception of their form. We are all familiar with basic geometric forms such as the circle, the square, the triangle. Our ability to recognize form allows us to assign meaning to it.

We associate the meaning of our experience to form. We talk about a circular argument, a square meal, and a love triangle. The ball-like shape of the fetal position conveys a different meaning from the broad erect stance of military posture. If you are feeling lonely, sad or dejected, the shape your body takes on is different from when you are elated. This is a good example of the relationship between function and expression, a theme we discussed in Chapter 2. Just as the two aspects of function and expression are actually one, so too are form and function. Form, function and expression are parts of the unified Whole.

The relationship of form and function is a chicken and egg puzzle. What comes first? Does form precede function or does function precede form? Did the form of our opposable thumbs lead to the creation and use of tools, or did our creation and use of tools lead to the form of opposable thumbs?

The form and function of our human anatomy are inseparable. If you change one, you change the other. A basic premise of holistic movement therapies is that the adaptability of the body can be incorporated to create positive change in mental and physical function. Dance Therapists frequently encourage clients to experience the changing shape of their body's moving form in order to elicit changes in mood.

Familiar Shape Forms

Do you know people who appear pin-like, with a narrow vertical posture? Perhaps you know someone wall-like who spreads into width. Familiar shapes, such as the wall, the ball, the pin, and the screw, are recognized forms of human posturing. These forms are also seen in archetypal renderings of the human shape, in everything from artistic sculpture to cartoon characters. Giacometti's sculptures portray humans in elongated pin-like forms. In contrast, Botero's art shows people as rotund and ball-like. Santa Claus characters are also typically ball-like.

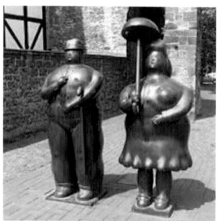

Ball-shaped sculpture by Botero

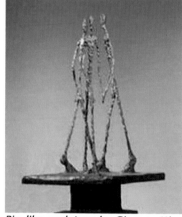

Pin-like sculpture by Giacometti

Familiar shapes are expressive and we attach meaning to them. However, the shape is the container for the meaning and is dependent on contexts and a multitude of other characteristics. For instance, Santa's ball-like appearance contributes to our interpretation of him as a jovial good-natured fellow. However, other ball-like representations, such as The Buddha and Jabba The Hut, can express different characteristics: from a state of serenity to malevolence. The wall-like character of Sponge Bob Square Pants does not convey the same meaning as the wall-like stance of soldiers permitted to stand "at ease".

In humans, these shapes are not simply due to anatomical considerations such as muscle, bone and fat. These are expressive shapes that are adopted and habitually maintained. Our habitual postural shapes reflect who we are.

Try this: In a standing position, take a wide stance and place your hands on your hips. Do you feel how this is characteristic of "Mister Clean" or "Peter Pan"? From this shape, drop your arms, cross one leg over the other and cross your arms over your chest. Let your body twist. Does this feel natural or unnatural? Who does this and when? A sulky teenager? A sultry starlet? An introspective poet? Now "come to attention", like a soldier. Bring your feet together underneath you, stand tall and pull your arms into your sides. Who does this shape serve and when?

The Shape of Body Attitude

Each one of us has a personal movement signature that is our home base. Part of this is recognizable in the shapes we frequent. Think about yourself and the postural stances you adopt. How do you tend to sit? Do you cross your legs? If so, do you cross them at the ankle or the knee? Do you cross the right over the left? How do you generally stand? Is your weight on both feet? Is your stance wide or narrow? Do your arms hang at your sides? Do you cross them or put your hands in your pockets? Are you more comfortable in the shape of a ball, a wall, a pin or a screw? Perhaps you adopt a habitual posture in which your upper body narrows and enfolds while your lower body supports you in a wide stance. In this pattern your upper body is more pin-like in contrast to your more wall-like lower body shape.

The shapes we inhabit are part of our Body Attitude, the home base to which we frequently return. In addition to the shapes we adopt, Body Attitude also includes patterns of preferences in body organization, space and dynamics. The Body Attitude of Marilyn Monroe included the indulging dynamic qualities of lingering in time and a delicate touch. She also incorporated a spiral shape in her poses. The next time you encounter someone you consider to be a forward thinker, see if you perceive a tendency to maintain a forward-ness in their Body Attitude.

Challenge yourself to become more aware of what characterizes your own personal movement signature: the shapes you form, the space you prefer, and the dynamic qualities that seem natural to you. How do these qualities serve you? Are there also circumstances in which your habits limit you?

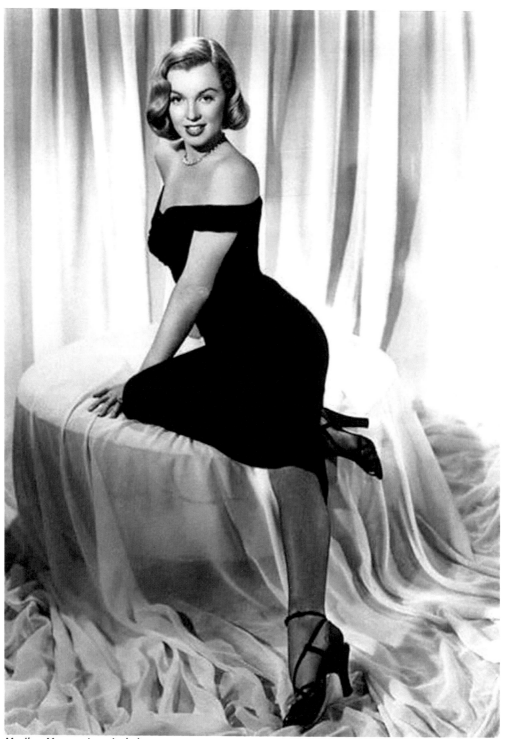

Marilyn Monroe in spiral shape

Moving our Shape - The Mode of Shape Flow

The meaningfulness of our moving shape develops as we develop. As infants, shape adjustments are all in relationship to self. These shape changes reflect how our body parts accommodate to the processes of function and expression as we breathe, suckle, defecate, cry, and burp. This process is the beginning of the emergence from undifferentiation to a sense of self.

The baseline of Shape Flow (described in Chapter 1) is an ongoing component of our body's changing shape. It is how we attend to ourselves and is present in how we prepare and recuperate. Whenever we remain in one position for too long, discomfort sets in, which tells us to re-position (move!). We do this twenty-four hours a day without thinking about it. So, part of a restful sleep includes rolling over and re-positioning ourselves throughout the night for maximum comfort. Someone who is comatose or experiencing diminished mobility while bed-ridden, runs the risk of developing bed sores due to inability to make continual Shape Flow adjustments.

Shape Flow examples include shifting your weight to find a new stance, rubbing a sore spot, licking your lips, twisting a strand of hair in thought, etc. Shape Flow reflects the body's intimate relationship with itself. Part of our socialization process includes the inhibition of overt Shape Flow. We are told as children, "stop fidgeting", "stop scratching" and "sit still". As adults, we associate the "inappropriate" use of Shape Flow with mental illness, disease, dysfunction or extreme emotional states. Repetitive self-soothing actions such as rocking and nail biting are commonly seen in these contexts.

While excessive Shape Flow can be evidence of dysfunction, diminished Shape Flow can also be problematic. Maintaining connection to our Shape Flow is an important part of our movement awareness. "Move it or lose it" is an adage that can be aptly applied to the movement of our Shape Flow. It is important to support our body's innate capacity for recuperation by noticing the cues we get to move. The next time you notice discomfort, before reaching for the pain relief medication, try stretching, shaking out and taking a deep breath. Allow your Shape to Flow!

Moving our Shape – The Mode of Bridging to the Environment

As babies learn to differentiate themselves from the world, they are motivated to connect to that world. They extend their arms to reach for, point to, and touch objects of interest. This is the process of creating, through movement, a bridge between themselves and the outer world. These movements are gestures that originate with the mover and are manifestations of the mover's intent directed outward to the world.

Bridging movements are an essential component in the building of communication skills. A clear example of this can be seen in policemen directing traffic. They use Spoke-like or Arc-like gestures to indicate where drivers should go. The airport personnel who direct aircraft to the gate communicate with the pilot through their Spoke-like or Arc-like gestures. The next time someone asks you for directions, observe how your gestures bridge to the space.

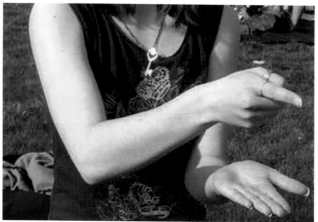

Gestural Directional movement

It is not just in isolated gestural actions that we spoke and arc. A karate kick requires full body involvement, as does inverting into a handstand. Both of these are bridging actions originating with the mover as they extend to make a connection outside of themselves.

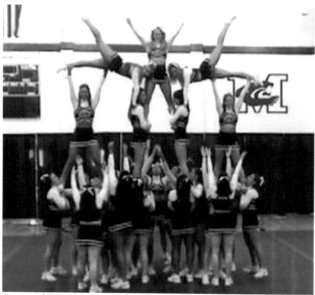

Postural Directional movement

The movement of our shape as it bridges to the environment reflects intent and attitude. Let's imagine two cheerleaders: Jean and Jill. Jean's cheering actions reflect her desire to connect to the world around her, specifically to members of her squad, the spectators and the team on the field. Jill however, appears to simply be going through the motions, with no intention beyond herself. Perhaps she has had a bad day or a fight with her boyfriend and is not invested in the cheerleading action. While both girls are moving the same body parts in the same spatial directions, it is clear that their movement is expressing something different. This example illustrates how we often interpret someone's conviction through movement. While Jean's cheering conveys conviction, Jill's does not.

Moving our Shape – The Mode of Molding and Adapting

Children love plush toys and stuffed animals. Have you ever thought about why this is so? The necessity to interact and coexist with things in our world is basic and underlies the capacity for our forms to adapt to the environment. Whether it is to pick up a spoon, wrap your hand around a tool or embrace a loved one, we are programmed to enjoy the experience of this adaptive ability. Children grasp, squeeze and hug their stuffed animals and find pleasure in the experience. We are wired for sensorial reward and seek things that make us feel good.

As we develop mentally and physically, we obtain pleasure by becoming masters over our ability to adapt and manipulate our environment, molding our shape to other shapes. It is this ability for adaptation that extends human potential and empowers us as individuals. The ability to mold to and hold a hammer enables a master carpenter to build a house. A carpenter and his tools become one. A loving embrace is an experience that helps two people become one. A concert violinist and her instrument seem to merge in the creation of beautiful music. These are all examples of the capacity of the human form to extend Self through molding and adapting to Other.

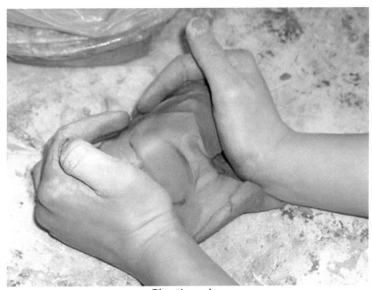

Shaping clay

The developmental movement progression is revealed through our shape as we move from oneness of Self to recognition of Other to a mutual interaction with Other. This is a progression that takes us from Shape Flow movements of tending to ourselves; to discovering and recognizing the world around us; to fully interacting and engaging with objects and people around us.

Just as developmental patterns of body organization occur in sequential stages (Chapter 6), so too, do the Modes of Shape Change described above. Although later stages of development are built on earlier stages, all stages are ever present and available to us as we move through our lives.

Shape Qualities – Change in the Core

We all observe and interpret the postural shapes we perceive. The next time you are looking at magazine ads, notice the postures the models adopt. How does the posture of a model selling perfume or clothing differ from the posture of the professional "expert" hawking medical or legal advice? These postures support the message of the advertisement.

How would you describe the shape of someone who appears to be depressed? Perhaps their chest is sunken and concave. In addition, there are other qualitative components present, such as the expression of energy as discussed in the previous chapter. Try this: adopt a concave sunken core body shape yourself and see what associations arise. From this posture, allow the core shape of your body to change. What did you do? Did you advance? Did you rise? Did you spread your torso? Did you do some combination of the above? As you made this core shape change, what, if anything, did your limbs do?

In the example above, it was possible to change your core shape without an overt change in the position of the limbs. However, as noted earlier, a change in any part changes the Whole. This is because relationships between Part/Whole have changed. In changing your core shape, the relationship between your core and your limbs has altered. There are endless possibilities for our Dynamic Alignment (Chapter 5).

Consider two different images. One is the snapshot taken as a competitive runner breaks through the finish line tape, chest advancing and arms thrown back at this moment of triumph. The other image, of a mother moving forward to embrace her child also involves the core advancing forward. But in this instance, her arms too are reaching forward toward her goal. While in both examples the core of the body is advancing, the core/limb relationship is different and in each case expresses the experience of the moment.

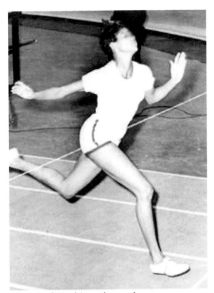

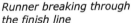
*Runner breaking through
the finish line*

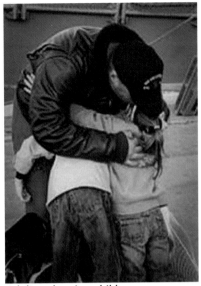
Adult embracing children

Affinities and Disaffinities between Shape and Space

In the two examples above, the body moves forward in the space. However, core shape change is not the same thing as directional intent in space. Space and Shape are two different components of movement. Consider the scenario of a reluctant child who is prodded to move forward to be embraced by an unfamiliar relative. While the child is moving forward, his reluctance may be seen in the fact that his core shape is actually retreating while his body as a Whole is moving forward. We are all familiar with the experience of the double message sent by the person embracing us with his arms while retreating with his core. This can be interpreted in a number of ways. Perhaps the person does not really want to embrace you. Perhaps they are being careful not to squeeze you too hard or crush your clothing.

Moving forward in space with an advancing core has a very different function and expression than moving forward in space while the core retreats. When the body as a Whole moves forward in the space supported by advancing in the core, there is an affinity between the space and the core shape change, contributing to a significant augmentation of the movement intent. When the core shape change contrasts with what the body is doing in space (the Whole body moving forward while the core retreats) the disaffinity expresses something very different. The same thing is true when moving upward in space supported by rising in the core (affined) versus moving upward in space while sinking in the core (disaffined). Try this: raise your hand upward in the space as if you were a student in a classroom trying to get the teacher's attention. Allow your core to rise in support of the arm gesture. Now, keep your arm up, but allow your core to sink. Notice how this core/gesture relationship changes the expression of the action.

Perhaps as you tried the above, your core also advanced while rising and then may have retreated while sinking. Try again: raise your hand, but this time while

101

rising in your core, add retreating as well. Are you able to do this? Now try keeping the arm up while sinking and advancing in the core. Could you feel how in each of the four variations:

core rising & advancing,   core sinking & retreating,

core rising & retreating,   core sinking & advancing

you became a different character, expressing a different meaning? Comedians and impersonators are intuitively skillful at embodying the subtleties and implications of core shape change.

Shape as Both Container and Content

Our language reflects the idea of shape as both mobile and stable. We talk about "shaping up" or "shaping" anything from topiaries to our retirement plans. We also talk about the shape of our nation's economy and the shape of things to come. This word play underscores our inherent understanding of the pattern of both change and constancy in the phenomenon of shape. We see the stable constant in shape, we also see the adaptable mobility of shape. The seemingly constant shapes of canyons and gorges are reflections of the mobile force of the rivers that carved them. In the same way, our living bone is shaped by the forces of our movement. A footprint is a shape created by the pressure of the body's weight moving against the ground.

Shapes express what shaped them. Shape is simultaneously expressive and functional. The interwoven connection between function and expression can be seen in all aspects of life. A sculptor's expression relies on the functionality of the tools and medium with which he is working. A chef shapes his particular haute cuisine through the interplay of his personal creative expression, as well as his functional knowledge of foods and cooking utensils. An architect's expression is bounded by the realities of the physical environment and the materials of construction.

The shape of EveryBody is an expression of the forces of our lives and the choices we have made. While we don't have control over our genetics, we can make changes in the adaptive shape of our bodies to enhance the function and expression of the contents and containers of our lives.

Chapter 11

The Expression of Space

Space has Meaning

Defining Space

The Kinesphere

The *Where* of Movement

Spatial Models

Moving in the Three Dimensions of Space

Moving in the Three Planes

Moving Three-Dimensionally

Spatial Awareness

Chapter 11

The Expression of Space

". . . the conventional idea of space as a phenomenon which can be separated from time and force and from expression, is completely erroneous."

"Space is a hidden feature of movement and movement is a visible aspect of Space." Rudolf Laban

Space has Meaning

Our spatial preferences and patterns are part of the Whole of our individual movement signature. Go to any public place and observe people as they walk. One person's posture may be very vertically erect with a buoyant bouncy walk. Perhaps another person has an obvious lumbering gait from side to side. A person in a hurry may lean forward toward his destination as he walks quickly. Part of the way we recognize people is our observation of their personal approach to space.

We generally think of space quantitatively. It is important to know where you are, where you are going and how much space is required. All of these reflect quantitative aspects of space. But space is also qualitative – it has meaning. Our metaphors of space clearly illuminate this. Think what it means to look up to a person or look down on someone. We are all aware when someone enters our personal space. This can be a positive or negative event depending on the relationship we have with that person, and the context of the situation. There are personal, social, cultural and gender aspects that are reflected in how we move through space. Qualitative aspects of space could also be thought of as psychological space. Our desire or need for space, the idea of personal territory, the sense of ownership of space, the feelings that different spaces elicit, all are part of the physio-socio-psychological character of space. Although there is plenty of literature about the use of personal space, our goal here is simply to help you become conscious of the space you choose to use.

You can begin by simply becoming aware of your feelings about space in different situations. For instance, how do you feel sitting in the middle seat of an airplane versus looking over a cliff's edge? How do you feel when gazing up at the stars or entering a cathedral? Our feelings about space color every aspect of daily life. Where do you choose to sit in a movie theater or classroom setting? Where is your place at the dinner table? What side of the bed do you sleep on? Now ask yourself why you have these spatial preferences. The container of space holds different meanings for different individuals. For example, choosing the window versus the aisle seat on an airplane reflects spatial preference. The person sitting by the window is gaining access to space outside of the plane. Conversely, the person sitting on the aisle may perceive he is gaining more access to the space inside of the plane. The space that we habitually inhabit reveals much about the nature of who we are.

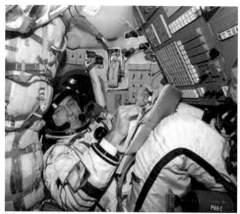 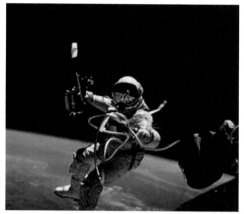

The container of space: confined to infinite

Defining Space

We identify space through the language labels we attach to it. We refer to outer space, we refer to personal space, and we say we need space (both literally and metaphorically). Through our language, we map our space, identifying location. Location can be as big an idea as "the next galaxy over", or as simple as "come sit next to me". In both of these examples, we understand space as a relative construct. Relationship and space are synonymous. How we define space reflects the basic pattern of duality: here/there, in/out, near/far, towards/away. All of these spatial dualities reflect the larger dualities of Part/Whole and Self/The World. The duality of Self/The World extends from our infinite concept of space to the space contained within our body.

The macro concepts of cosmic space are in the realms of physics and theology. We, however, are going to explore space relative to the daily experience of the moving human body. We can start by defining the space through which we move. According to Rudolf Laban, "Space is a hidden feature of movement, and movement is a visible aspect of space". For example, if I direct you to "stand behind me", you are only able to do this relative to both bodies involved. Your front is facing my back. If I turn and face you, the space is the same, but our spatial *relationship* is different. We primarily perceive and interpret space through the form of our bodies. In Laban's system of Movement Analysis, space is defined and codified from the body perspective. While space theory can seem abstract (associations occur with geometry and theoretical constructs) we encourage you to stay with it, because understanding space can reveal much about our movement preferences, patterns and potential.

In Laban's system, we identify the large container of space (the world of our environment) as general space. General space is the space we travel through; down the street, through the woods, over the mountain. The personal bubble of space is our kinesphere. The kinesphere is defined by the extent of our reach, and is the space through which we gesture, work and play. The space contained within our body is our inner space. Inner space is defined by all the space within us: a full or empty belly, the space between cells, the space occupied by all that is contained inside our skin.

106

The Kinesphere

Contained within the larger environment of the general space, we each have a bubble of personal space that surrounds us called the Kinesphere. The roots of this word are "kinesis" for movement and "sphaira" for ball or globe. It is literally the sphere in which our movement occurs. It is defined as the space we can access without taking a step to a new place. Our personal reach space, the Kinesphere, stays with us as we travel through the general space. Remember that actions that don't shift our weight to a new location or change our body position to a new place are called gestures. Gestures are actions of a single body part, like a wave of the hand.

Within the Kinesphere, we can delineate meaningful zones of movement. These zones are based on the size of our gestures and may be categorized as Near-reach, Mid-reach and Far-reach space. The use of our reach space is both functional and expressive. For instance, when hailing a cab, fully extending your arm in space can get the driver's attention. Pulling into Near-reach space while lowering your voice may assist you in dealing with a timid child. Many task related gestures, like washing dishes and hammering a nail are best accomplished in Mid-reach space. Imagine how the meaning of space changes when meeting someone and you reach to shake his hand. More often than not, handshakes take place in the Mid-reach space. Use of the extremes of reach space change the meaning of the movement. If you barely extend your hand, keeping it close to yourself, it has a very different meaning than if you reach out to the full extent.

Movement is a complex event, so remember that reach space is just one part of the bigger picture. In this example, the Near-reach handshake pulls the two individuals closer together, which can feel intimate or invasive, welcoming or off-putting. In the Far-reach handshake, a fully extended arm can be interpreted as open and inviting or as a way to set a boundary (keeping one's opponent at arm's length).

Use of our reach space is one of the many expressive aspects of movement. Performers often make use of extremes for theatrical impact. Just as in a monologue, the actor can enhance meaning by varying his voice from a whisper to a shout, his gestures have the potential to change meaning as he moves from small contained gestures to those that are fully extended in space. Try this: Imagine giving someone the "thumbs up" gesture as a sign of approval. First try this close to your body in near reach space. Then move the gesture to mid reach space. Finally, extend your arm fully to give the 'thumbs up" in far reach space. Can you see how a change of reach space alters the meaning of the gesture within a specific context? In terms of our own personal expressiveness, we tend to inhabit comfort zones. In addition to functional and contextual aspects of reach space, some people prefer to extend themselves further into their Kinesphere than others do. Where do you see this in yourself and in others? The next time you are in a group setting, see if you can notice how people are using their Kinespheres.

The *Where* of Movement

We have defined space as the relationship between ourselves and the environment through which we move. The space of where you are going is relative to the space where you are coming from. Just as we mostly take our bodies for granted, we take the space through which we move mostly for granted, until we need more or less of it, or require directions. The relationship between our biological form and the space of our environment is a given of our existence. Movement occurs in space and space reveals movement. Try this: point your finger to something directly in front of you. Note what that something is. Now drop your arm and make a quarter turn of your body. Point again to the same thing you did before. You should notice that in the first case, you were pointing forward and in the second case you were pointing sideward. This is an example of the fact that our body determines spatial relationship.

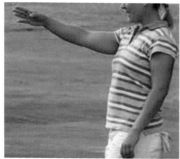 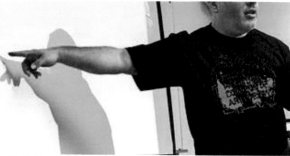

Pointing forward   *Pointing sideways*

Our conception of space and direction comes from our experience of our bodies. We stand upright in line with the pull of gravity, so we understand "up" and "down" in relation to gravity. Inside the container of our torso, our Diaphragm moves "up" and "down" as we breathe "in" and "out". We stand "up" and sit "down". We climb "up" a ladder to paint the ceiling and climb back "down" to scrub the floor. We rise to the occasion and fall down on the job.

The structure of our bodies is how we understand "right" from "left". We are bilaterally symmetrical with two lungs and two kidneys, two eyes and two ears, two arms, and two legs (among other body parts!). The wiring of our brain causes us to experience one of our "sides" as being more dominant. Although we may not think about it much, part of our self-identity includes being either right or left handed. Ice skaters, gymnasts and divers have a clear preference for turning either right or left. Their training takes this preference into account and is part of the equation in attaining higher levels of mastery. In America, we drive on the "right" side of the road. In Britain, they drive on the "left" side of the road. In a dispute, one can take a side or see both sides.

We experience the front and back of ourselves because of the placement of our eyes, nose and mouth, and the way in which our anatomy is designed to carry us through space. We lean "forward" to smell a rose and recoil "backward" from a rotten odor. All of our vehicles of transportation are designed to move us forward in space, reflecting our form. When you go for a drive, it is understood that you are driving forward. When you go for a walk, it is understood that you are not walking backward! We move forward with a plan, or we back off and head in another direction.

The experience of up/down, side/side and front/back creates the three-dimensional experience of ourselves. While our bodies always occupy the three dimensions of height, width and depth, we can (and do) choose to move one, two or three dimensionally in space. A map of the body (such as the location of boney landmarks in relationship with each other) lets us know **what** is moving. A map of Space lets us know **where** we are moving. While space is infinite, we can identify spatial landmarks that create a metaphorical "skeleton of space". Just as knowledge of the inner architecture of our skeleton contributes to awareness of movement, knowledge of the architecture of space also enhances our awareness of movement.

Spatial Models

Although models of space are generally based on our body – there are different perspectives of Space. Some are fixed, like room organization. Some models are ever changing – "to the right" will depend on where you are. For example, in a group exercise class, the instructor may tell you to move to the right. But – does she mean to the right of your body, or to the right side of the room? They could be in opposite directions! In the language of theater, stage space is from the perspective of the performers, not the audience. Stage right is based on the actor's right as he faces the audience. When his back is to the audience, stage right is now to his left! Upstage is the area furthest away from the audience and downstage is the space closest to the audience. The terms "upstage" and "downstage" are holdovers from early theater history when stages were slanted (raked). The actor was actually moving uphill when moving away from the audience and downhill when approaching the audience.

The model of space we are using was codified by Rudolf Laban, who created a system for describing and analyzing human movement. Laban observed people moving in work, play, dance, martial arts and communal ritualized activities. In this model, space is designated from the perspective of the mover. Right is always the right side of the body, and up is always over the mover's head aligned with the length of the body. So, in this spatial map, when one is lying down, "up" is toward the head rather than toward the ceiling. The mover's body is the spatial key in mapping our movement.

Moving in the Three Dimensions of Space

Try this: swing your arm freely in the space around you. Let it go this way and that, every which way. If you tried to describe each and every point in space that your arm moved through, it would be like counting grains of sand on the beach. While space has infinite directions, we start by identifying three dimensions of space: our height, our width and our depth. Each dimension maps a pull in space, which can be thought of as a line having two equal and opposite directions. Start from up and down, which gives us the dimension of height. Try this: with your arms hanging by your sides, direct them straight upwards. Note – do not swing them forward, let them spoke upward, keeping them close to the body. Return them back to where they started, moving along the same pathway. Your movement has occurred in the two directions of the Vertical dimension - up and down. This dimension is derived from gravity and our upright stance. We also assign meanings of power along this dimension and historically have located Heaven as "up above" and Hell as "down below".

The dimension of our depth is a line composed of the two directions of forward and backward, the two directions of the Sagittal dimension. Try this: put your palms together at your navel. Move your hands directly forward, then return them to your center along the same path. Our sense of front and back is derived from the design of our legs to move us forward, and the location of our face (particularly our eyes). We extend our physical reality to associations with time, in which the future lies in front of us and the past is behind us.

The dimension of our width is a line composed of the two sideward directions of right and left. Try this: place your right hand on your belly and move it across your body to the left and continue to spoke out into left side space. Move your arm as far as it will go in this dimension without twisting into it. Return along the same path and try to unfold the arm along a straight line to the right side of your body. Take care not to rotate the body or turn your head to watch your hand travel. This movement has occurred in the Horizontal Dimension, which is derived from our bilateral symmetry. The meaningfulness of side-ed-ness becomes extended to such things as political thought, in which beliefs are frequently identified as leaning to the right or left.

The design and three-dimensional volume of the human body restricts our capacity for pure movement along one dimension. However it is possible, at least in some sense, to move in one dimension. Some examples of one-dimensional movement are: jumping straight up in the air (Vertical Dimension), pushing an elevator button directly in front of you (Sagittal Dimension), clapping your hands (Horizontal Dimension). One-dimensional movement can be simple, and it also can be very powerful in its clarity. Both ballet and the martial arts call upon the power of one-dimensional movement. We have identified three dimensions, each one having two equal opposite directions, for a total of six one-dimensional directions in our map of space. These are: up, down, right, left, forward, backward.

Moving in the Three Planes

Two-dimensional movement is movement occurring in a plane. Just as there are three dimensions, there are three planes. Planal movements combine two dimensions and leave out the third. The axis of rotation for each of the planes is its missing dimension. Metaphors for the three planes are a door for the Vertical Plane, a wheel for the Sagittal Plane, and a table for the Horizontal Plane. Can you see how each of these metaphors is a reflection of the form and function of the human body?

Try this: do a typical Jumping Jack. This is a movement in the door plane (also called the Vertical Plane) which utilizes the up/down and right/left aspects of the body. Actions of the arms and legs in this plane are defined as the anatomical actions of abduction (away from the body's midline) and adduction (toward the body's midline). Jumping Jacks are a pure example of Vertical Plane movement. Envision doing Jumping Jacks in a doorway, and you can see how the action occurs in this plane. Movement in the door plane has a flat quality because it has no depth. The four directions of the Vertical Plane are: up/right, up/left, down/right, and down/left. Now try this: stand with your body forming a big "X". Note that *vertical* each hand and foot is placed at the corners of this plane. Next, pull your hands and feet together reaching purely up/down in the Vertical dimension. Spread your arms back to the corners of the Door Plane. Notice how they have maintained their "upness" in space while adding "sidedness". Your arms have moved from a one-dimensional pull through space to a two-dimensional pull through space. In other words, you have moved from the Vertical Dimension to the Vertical Plane. The dimension and the plane share the same name of Vertical because the up/down directions are dominant. Like a door, our model for the planes is rectangular rather than square. Rectangular forms are reiterated in many spatial designs, from our architecture to a standard paper size. When moving through the Vertical Plane, the long side of the rectangle is the primary aspect of Space, while the short side is the secondary aspect of space.

Try this: stand as though you are preparing to bowl a strike. In this position one leg is in front of the other and your body is inclining forward. Starting with *→ bowl* the arm behind you to prepare, swing the arm forward in an arc as though releasing the ball. This is an example of an action in the wheel plane, also called the Sagittal Plane. The wheel plane has both depth and height. Movement in this plane rolls us and swings us backwards and forwards through space. A jogger in the park is moving through the wheel plane; running forward while his arms and legs swing forward and back. The anatomical actions emphasized in this plane are flexion (bending or folding) and extension (unfolding, straightening). The Sagittal Plane combines the dimensions of forward/backward and up/down, but is missing the right/left dimension. A somersault is a good example of movement that also occurs within the wheel plane. The four directions of the wheel plane (or Sagittal Plane) are: forward/up, forward/down, backward/up, backward/down. Try this: lunge forward on one leg, keeping the other leg extended behind you. Slightly incline the torso forward and reach the arms up and forward. While keeping one arm where it is, sweep the other arm over the head to the backward/up corner of *→ sagittal* this plane. Try to remain facing front as you do this.

You may experience the difficulty of forming an "X" shape in this plane. This is due to both our anatomy and our habitual patterns. Access to the space behind us is somewhat limited but also frequently under-utilized. The structure of our joints and the placement of our eyes emphasize the space in front of us. However, due to our life styles and technology, this forward emphasis has further hampered our ability to move in the space behind us. Think about the typical office desk chair. The chair can easily move backward on its coasters. We can the chair's movement to move us backward, rather than our own movement! While this has advantages, it is just one simple example of how we limit our own capacity for movement in all directions. Our language reflects the experience of the difficulty of accessing the back space. We speak of bending over backwards for someone when we go beyond what is expected. The Sagittal Plane and the Sagittal Dimension are named the same because forward and backward are the primary directions.

The table plane has both width and depth, but no up/down aspect of space. Moving the hips to use a hula hoop, twisting to looking behind you, or reaching to the corners of a table are some examples of movement in the table plane, also called the Horizontal Plane. The anatomical action of rotation is characteristic of this plane. The four directions of the table or Horizontal Plane are: right/forward, left/forward, right/backward and left/backward. Try this: reach your right arm right and forward at the level of your navel (as if you are reaching to the far corner of a big table). Keep your right arm reaching toward this goal, but add your left arm reach to the other forward corner of the table. Now- lift your left leg to the level of the left/backward corner while balancing on the other leg. If you can do this (hooray!) you are now reaching to three of the four corners of the Horizontal Plane. A more common movement example occurring in this plane is reaching for something in the back right passenger seat as you drive. In addition to reaching actions of the limbs, this plane also frequently involves twisting actions (rotation) of the spine. In the above example, notice that your spine supports the reach of the arm backward by rotating to the right. The Horizontal Plane has the Horizontal Dimension (right/left) as the primary pull in space.

horizontal

To summarize, each plane has four directions, one for each corner. This gives us a total of twelve planal directions in our spatial map. Add these twelve directions to the six one-dimensional directions we named earlier, and we have a total of eighteen of the twenty-six possible directions in the Laban model of space.

Moving Three-Dimensionally

So what, you may be asking, are the final eight directions? These directions each combine all three dimensions, and can be envisioned as the corners of a cube. Try this: go back to the Door Plane for a moment. Reach your right arm up and to the right corner of this Vertical Plane. This spatial direction has width and height, but no depth. Keep your arm up and right, but add the forward direction, as if you were moving to the front/high corner of a cube. Try to equalize the directional pulls so you are equally up, equally right, and equally forward. The addition of depth to width and height gives a sense of three-dimensional volume in space. Just as a plane is a model for two-dimensional movement, we use the model of a cube for three-dimensional movement.

Visualize yourself standing in the center of a cube. If the room you are in is relatively square shaped, this is easy to do. Try this: point to the right/forward/high corner of the cube - where two adjacent walls and the ceiling meet. Notice the three spatial pulls of this corner. Now sweep your arm across to the other side, directing it to the left/forward/ high corner of your cube. From here move to the back/high corners of the cube. Keep going in this circuit around the top of the cube until you return to where you started. The remaining four directions in the cube are its low corners. Change all of the upward directions to downward directions and you have mapped the bottom of the cube.

Using the Laban model of space, we name the eight corners of the cube the Diagonal Directions. Although we have identified eight Diagonal Directions, there are only four Diagonals. Just like the dimensions, which each have two equal and opposite directions, each Diagonal also has two equal and opposite directions. Try this: reach one arm to the right/forward/high corner of the cube. Using the same arm, move to the opposite corner (left/backward/low) along the most direct pathway. Notice that you have moved through the center of the cube. Earlier we stayed on the surface of the cube as we traced the upper corners. To move along any of the four Diagonals, you must pass through the center of the cube. See if you can identify the other three Diagonals in the cube.

Previously, we addressed the fact that there are different spatial maps. Everyday usage of the term "diagonal" does not always include three dimensions. In our map, it does. This goes back to the fact that our body is the key to our spatial map. The contralateral movement pattern (the basis of human locomotion) combines up/down, forward/back and right/left directions, fully utilizing the body's three-dimensional volume.

Pure Diagonal movement is the most complex, requiring combined joint actions of: flexion/extension with abduction/adduction with right/left rotation. In contrast to the simplicity of Dimensional movement and the flatness of Planal movement, Diagonal movement has a more voluminous feel.

Spatial Awareness

The true three-dimensionality of the moving human body comes from our ability to change among one, two or three-dimensional spatial pulls. We can choose the purity and clarity of a one-dimensional thrust. We can spread our form along a two-dimensional plane or spiral along a Diagonal. Where we choose to move in space, as well as where we choose **not** to move, has both functional and expressive implications.

Becoming aware of your space is a first step in clarifying movement – whether it is to perfect an athlete's jump shot, coach an actor in a specific character role, or re-pattern an inefficient movement habit. Clarifying space helps us to fulfill our movement goals. We are conscious of space when aiming a dart or parking a car, but generally our movement through space is not something we register consciously. Remember the last time you moved through a crowd of people – collisions were fairly infrequent! We have the innate ability to navigate our bodies, but bringing our conscious awareness to the space we move through helps us to organize our body more efficiently.

Becoming aware of space is a fundamental aspect of movement awareness. The functional and expressive components of space are a part of the bigger Whole that is human movement. Space is not just a theoretical construct. It is a tangible experience made visible through our movement. As we jump ahead, fall back or side step an issue, the body/space relationship is constantly available to us.

Where we move our bodies in space creates boundaries, connections, extensions, and possibilities – all of which has significance. Space both contains and frees EveryBody.

Chapter 12

Awareness Leading to Transformation

Connecting Everything

Problematic Patterns

Movement Re-education

Body Language: The Facts and the Fiction

Coming Full Circle

Chapter 12

Awareness Leading to Transformation

"Our bodies remember wholeness in the midst of fragmentation"
Terry Tempest Williams

Connecting Everything

Understanding the Whole requires a systematic identification and analysis of the parts. That's what we have attempted to do in the preceding chapters, by identifying the parts of movement. The ultimate objective however, is to re-integrate the parts that together form the Whole of human movement. In order to become consciously aware of movement, it was necessary in the previous chapters to dissect movement for detailed discussion. However, all aspects of movement, which we have identified as the *what* of Body, the *how* of Dynamics, the container of Shape, and the *where* of Space, are constantly and intimately connected into the Whole of our movement. A change in one aspect of movement can result in change in other aspects of movement. In other words, a change of a part changes the Whole. Everything is connected.

It is this phenomenon of the interconnectedness of parts that distinguishes the authors' practice, **WholeMovement** and Laban/Bartenieff Movement Studies from many other types of somatic practices. **WholeMovement** does not address a symptom in isolation. In fact, the symptom itself may actually be of minimal significance when trying to get to the source of an issue. The authors' approach to maximizing movement potential includes a consideration of habits and preferences in body organization and shape, spatial tendencies and patterns of dynamics and phrasing.

Every individual, from genetic make-up, personal history and life experience, has a personal movement signature, which is as unique to that individual as their handwriting. Bringing a person into increased awareness of their unconscious movement choices allows them to optimize their movement potential. While we all have access to a wide range of movement possibilities, lack of awareness of our unconscious habits can lead to an imbalance. Rather than attempting to change movement preferences, it is important to be aware of the full range of choices available. This leads to more successful movement choices, rather than remaining limited by unconscious habits. A benefit of this approach to change is that it can begin from any body organization, spatial direction, dynamic configuration or shape mode. There is more than one inroad to change. For example, a **WholeMovement** session might entail working with an individual to increase their awareness of how they use space, which could have beneficial results in body organization or dynamic range.

Problematic Patterns

While advancements in science and technology have led to improvements in life quality, they also have the capacity to diminish a high quality of life. The largest of these is the removal of the depth and range of our moment-to-moment experience of our moving bodies. While most of us no longer need to use full postural exertion to make a living, the problem that results is that we become less able to move with full postural mobility. If you don't use it, you lose it. We go to the gym or schedule physical activities in an attempt to compensate, but this does not solve the problem. We tone our abs, we increase cardio-vascular endurance, we strengthen our quads, we stretch our hamstrings, but once again we all too often are addressing parts in isolation and miss the big picture of enhancing full-bodied function and expression.

In too much of contemporary life, full-bodied movement is not only unnecessary, it is frankly discouraged. Starting with telling our children "don't fidget", to traveling everywhere by car and spending countless hours in front of the TV or computer screen, our ability to move freely and expressively is compromised. It would be extremely beneficial for passengers on a long plane flight to have the freedom to stand up, fully extend their bodies, shake out and vocalize. Unfortunately, not only is this impractical, it would be judged as odd and an infringement of the personal space of others.

Think of some of the common problematic patterns we see in daily life: lower back pain, tension headaches and eyestrain, Carpal Tunnel Syndrome, Irritable Bowel Syndrome, sleep disturbances, etc. These maladies are frequently seen as inevitable results of aging. We propose that this is a fallacy and that many of these "inevitable" problems could be alleviated, or even eliminated, by developing an aware practice of movement. While awareness is the first part of the process, it has to be connected to an ongoing daily physical practice. Don't worry, we are not talking here about arranging to spend time on the treadmill, hiring a personal trainer or signing up for yoga classes (although these may be beneficial activities).

What we are advocating is a mindful approach to movement in all of life's daily activities. Remember, you can choose to take the stairs rather than the elevator. You could park your car further away and take the opportunity to walk and connect to the pleasure and sensation of moving your body. When you get dressed in the morning, do you sit down to put on your socks? Is this because it's hard to keep your balance while standing on one leg? Recognizing that your balance is compromised in this activity, perhaps you could then choose to practice standing on one leg while doing another activity, like brushing your teeth. We often diminish movement without being aware of it. Increasing your awareness of your movement choices leads to a more mindful approach to life, health and well-being.

One can rarely open a newspaper without seeing a report on the plague of chronic back pain. Remedies and interventions run the gamut from over the counter pain medications to physical therapy, back braces and the ultimate – immobilization of the spine through surgery. Chronic back pain is, more often than not, a symptom that results from movement patterns that have been present for months, if not years. Someone whose job requires a long commute by car, followed by long hours sitting at a computer, is ripe for developing a chronic back pain condition. Emphasis on treating the symptom will have limited success, but seems to be the primary focus in most modes of treatment. Once again, an isolated symptom is a very small piece of our total being. A successful treatment of a chronic condition such as back pain, requires a consideration of the person as a Whole. The person with a long commute who sits at the computer all day could benefit from small changes that would help them to recuperate. Changing sitting positions, taking short breaks to stand up and walk around, rolling the shoulders, stretching, changing eye focus to attend to the larger environment, are just a few examples of changes that might interrupt the imbalance of the work pattern that leads to chronic back pain.

Wholeness rests in balancing the patterns of exertion and recuperation, the interplay between our inner and outer worlds, and the relationship between action and stillness, being and doing. It is lack of awareness which leads to imbalance in the above rhythms of life, and eventually can result in injury or disease. Awareness is an ongoing process of continuing education about ourselves and communication with ourselves. The process of education promotes human development, which is about growth and change. Just as education doesn't stop with the attainment of a formal degree, movement education is a lifelong, ongoing process that requires continual re-investment. As practitioners of **WholeMovement**, our goal is to facilitate this ongoing process of growth and development.

Movement Re-education

Just as we encourage children to plan for their future through education, we can encourage children to be mindful of their moving bodies to ensure health and well-being as they move through life. The process of aging does not have to be one of diminished mobility and pain. As movers we continue to change. The motive of trying to "maintain" one's level of fitness or "reverse" the aging process misses the point. It is an "all or nothing" approach. Movement itself is change. Why should we assume that we continue to move in the same way throughout the course of our lives? Embracing movement potential in every phase of life sets the course for continued renewal and revitalization for the Whole of the life cycle.

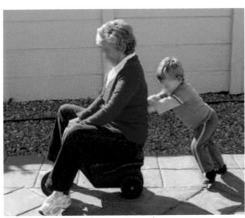 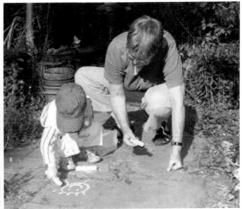

Old and young playing together

We would be better served to change the way we think about movement generally. Rather than regarding it as something "added on" or extra-curricular, we should remind ourselves that movement is the foundation of our existence. We could say that movement is as important as breathing and eating, but both of those are only possible through movement!

To increase your consciousness of your moving body, begin by making the decision to attend to your movement. When you find yourself standing in line at the grocery store, rather than thinking ahead to what is next on your agenda for the day, be present in the moment and become aware of how you are standing. Is your weight balanced on one foot or two? Are you seeing what's around you, or not? Be aware of your breathing, allowing yourself to fully experience the process. When moving through daily routines such as getting in and out of a car, become aware of how you are accomplishing this functionally. How do you position your arms when conversing with someone? Do they hang loosely at your sides, do you clasp your hands in front of you, do your fold you arms across your chest? How do you routinely stand, sit, walk? Observe how your patterns are similar or different from the patterns of others.

As you become more movement conscious, you will become more familiar with the constant Shape Flow adjustments that you make throughout the day as you check-in and recuperate. We urge you to more fully experience and explore this ongoing monologue of your body. You might be surprised by how much better you feel when you consciously experience and amplify the previously unconscious movements of self. On the other hand, you may also become conscious of tensions and irritations that you feel. Once you recognize discomfort you can move in ways to become more comfortable.

We sometimes learn to deaden sensation as a protection against discomfort and pain. While this pattern begins in order to serve us, it can become a habit that diminishes us. You can choose to ignore hunger, fatigue, a crick in your neck, a pain in your back, if you are working against a deadline in a high stress situation. The ability to ignore discomfort can be a good thing in some situations. However, if this practice is repeated often enough, the consequences can be severe. A habit of cutting off sensation leads to loss of movement awareness. Before you can find release from tension or chronic pain, you must first become aware that tension and chronic pain are present. This is an important step in transforming from a condition of discomfort to one of ease.

While we have the capacity to enjoy the pleasures of sensation through the foods we eat, and the sights, sounds, scents and textures with which we surround ourselves, more often than not, our body awareness is limited to the extremes of pain or pleasure. We lose recognition of the subtle sensations of our ongoing movement life. By reawakening our awareness and becoming mindful of our moving selves, we find more access to balance in the constantly changing continuums of Function/Expression, Mobility/Stability, Inner/Outer and Exertion/Recuperation. The process of balancing these dualities moves us towards Wholeness.

Body Language: The Facts and the Fiction

Let's think back to the beginning of the book where we define movement. We noted how difficult this was, due to the all-encompassing, omnipresent nature of movement. It is the sea in which we swim, and so much the fabric of our existence, that we are largely unaware of it. We are constantly observing and monitoring movement on both conscious and unconscious levels, and responding based on the information we perceive. We are always interpreting movement. For example, a person standing with his arms folded across his chest may be interpreted by a so-called body language expert as being "closed off". In actuality there are any number of credible interpretations, and more information is required. The person might be feeling chilly, covering a stain on his shirt, or perhaps, folding his arms in a habit that helps that individual to connect to himself and to concentrate.

A person's non-verbal communication has universal aspects, but there are also cultural patterns, as well as patterns that are unique to each individual. Any interpretation of "Body Language" requires knowledge of the context in which movement is occurring and an awareness of one's own preferences and patterns which color our interpretations.

We are all programmed to be observers of movement. Because we are social beings, we have to be able to successfully interact with others and interpret the movement of others. To make this point, the authors often use the following experience in their movement classroom:

The experience starts with students pairing up for a mirroring exercise (many of you may have done this on some occasion). Facing each other, one partner leads while the other follows along, attempting to move in synchrony with the leader. While this may seem to be simply a matter of visual tracking, other modes of the perceptual process are also at work, including the kinesthetic sense. Our understanding of another's movement is based in our experience of our own movement. Skilled movers, due to their developed movement intuition, are often able to achieve such successful synchrony that neither they, nor those observing, are able to tell who is leading and who is following. The point of the exercise is to move in unison with your partner. Everyone can have success with this experience. In the next step, a third party is added. The leader now stands behind the follower. The third person watches the leader and verbally instructs the follower in how to move.

The results are often hilarious. This is due to the fact that language is linear and the meaning unfolds one word at a time, whereas the gestalt of a movement allows for many parts to be understood simultaneously. We have been fascinated to note that the translation process is much more successful when the translator uses an image – such as "move your arms like a bat" or "move as though you are praying". The process really falls apart when the translator tries to describe the action of every body part.

The above exercise is generally very effective in illustrating how much we unconsciously communicate non-verbally, the shortcomings of translating movement into words, and how skilled we all are as observers and interpreters of the subtleties of movement (although we are not always aware of it). Even a self-described "non-mover" has no difficulty picking up such details as palm facing, level of muscular tension and timing.

It is built into the human condition to be perceptive of movement. This ability is what allows humans to interact and work communally. Movement reflects the culture of its origin. That is why ballet looks the way it does, that is why hip-hop looks the way it does. These dance forms embody the values of the culture which produced them. In this case, the experience and values of the French aristocracy versus the experience and values of inner city youth reflect the context from which these dances developed. Cultural movement values are seen in everyday expression as well as in codified dance forms. Think about the common characterization of Italians as being flamboyant in their use of gestures, or the characterization of New Englanders as being physically reserved. This is why one must take any simplistic and reductionist interpretation of "Body Language" with a huge grain of salt!

We are all moving all the time. We all take in and give out movement information all the time, whether we are conscious of it, or not. Like the connective tissue that connects all the structures of our bodies to form a Whole being, movement is the connective tissue that forms the Whole of existence, from the unique individual experience to the shared cultural experience, to the universal human experience.

Coming Full Circle

In analyzing movement, we have broken it down into component parts: The Body (*what* is moving), Space (*where* we are moving), Dynamic Qualities (*how* we are moving) and Shape (the form our body adopts). We have talked about the architecture of the human body with its skeleton, muscle and organs. We discussed the organization of body parts and the concepts of Breath Support, Core Support and Rotation. We discussed concepts of Space, as we mapped the three-dimensionality of our world and how our body structure both defines, and is defined through, its spatial characteristics. We also addressed the qualities of expression which characterize the dynamic range of human movement, from a delicate touch to packing a punch. We spoke about how the body shapes its form relative to itself and its environment.

All of these pieces form the larger picture that is human movement. We all are expressive bodies with the same basic structure, moving through Space on planet Earth. The movement components of Body, Space, Dynamics and Shape do not exist in isolation. They form an integrated Whole. For example, we observe a charismatic person making a speech. Think about the ways we would describe him: confident, poised, regal, inspiring, powerful. Now think about how his movement leaves us with these impressions: his vertical upright posture, direct focus, how he uses articulate gestures to connect to others and drive home the points he is making, the rhythm and phrasing of his delivery, etc. The constellation of the mover's body organization, spatial intent and dynamic range is what leads the observer to an interpretation.

The process of analysis allows for identification and clarification by breaking a Whole into its component parts. However, the goal of analysis is a synthesis of the Whole. Don't forget, the Whole is greater than the sum of its parts. The synthesis of the Whole of movement is seeing and understanding how the parts are related to the Whole.

Becoming conscious of your moving self requires mindfulness of the sensations of your body, the support of Space, and accessing a broad range movement expression. The benefit is increased freedom from the limitations of unconscious habitual patterns. Movement patterning is to some degree innate, for instance reflexes and developmental patterns are built into the human design. However, personal movement choices are selected because they make sense at the time and serve us in some way. These movements become habits through repetition. Over time some of these choices may no longer be functionally efficient. For instance, if you sprain your ankle, you might compensate by shifting more of your weight to your other foot. While this choice initially serves to minimize pain and allows the injury to heal, if the pattern is maintained long after the injury has healed, you have set yourself up for other possible injuries arising from the imbalance.

Revisiting movement choices that we made earlier in our lives helps us to reassess the benefit of them in our current lives. The expressive aspects of our movement also involve choice and change over time. You probably don't wear the same clothing you wore in high school (not just because it no longer fits you), because it no longer "suits" who you are today.

The nature of the Whole rests in the active ongoing process of the balance of opposites. We need to be both mobile and stable. We need to know when to go with the flow and when to stand firm. We need to know when to let go and when to hang on.

We benefit from attending to the inner sensations of our body. Recognizing the sensations of both pleasure and pain is vital to our well-being. We are encouraged to ignore pain and overindulge in pleasure – with unfortunate results. We benefit from finding balance between our inner world and our outer world, where we meet challenges, search for meaning and interact with others.

It is essential to understand the interwoven connection between function and expression. Many of our perceived vicious cycles are related to a disconnection between the two sides of this one coin. For example, someone who is feeling down will not be motivated to get up and out. They are likely to just sink further into immobility and depression.

We need to understand the true nature of patterns of exertion and recuperation. Taking a vacation may not be recuperation. Working hard at something may not be exertive. Balance in the rhythm of exertion and recuperation is necessary – daily, weekly, monthly, yearly and over the Whole course of our lives.

Balance in the dualities of life (Stability/Mobility, Inner/Outer, Function/Expression and Exertion/Recuperation) lies in increasing our awareness of the moving body. Our awareness of ourselves as bodies, through our movement, has the potential to lead to transformation.

EveryBody has a body, EveryBody *is a Body.*

Authors' Epilogue

The *WholeMovement* Approach

Movement is the most basic experience of life. It is how we interact with the world around us. We all share the experience of a moving body, but each one of us has a unique movement signature. Our personal movement signature reveals who we are in how we move. The authors' *WholeMovement* experiential approach to body education discovers and utilizes this personal uniqueness in order to maximize movement potential and decrease discomfort from stress and chronic pain. The process of addressing the Wholeness of the mover increases the sense of overall well-being.

WholeMovement is different from other movement practices in that it is closer to the phenomenon of movement itself, which is multi-faceted, multi-layered, complex and pervades all aspects of life. Other movement practices generally compartmentalize, focusing on specific discreet aspects of movement such as: cardio-vascular fitness, aesthetics, stress reduction, and physical technique. In the practice of *WholeMovement* principles are applied according to the specific needs and preferences of the mover and the context of their life, rather than a prescriptive "one size fits all" approach.

The philosophy of *WholeMovement* embraces movement as a life-long ongoing process, rather than something we lose as we age. Because movement is change, we coach to increase ongoing resilience and adaptability. The objective is to allow movers to gain skills for their own transformation, empowering each individual to be their own best resource. When a client experienced in the practice of *WholeMovement* works with other movement professionals (coaches, therapists, chiropractors, teachers) he is better able to utilize what those practitioners have to offer.

Although movement is a complex process, a very simple change (such as awareness of breath support) can lead to more profound life changes. Remember that a change in any part results in a change of the Whole, as the following story illustrates.

Laura's Story

Many years ago, while participating in a movement class, we were instructed to vocalize a series of vowel sounds to increase awareness of breath. Suddenly, I became short of breath and strangely anxious. I couldn't tolerate the sound around me. I felt impatient and angry and there was a black frame around my field of vision. I felt something large, dark and terrifying rising from my depths and I knew I had to escape before it erupted. I ran from the studio in a blind panic to the furnace room – the farthest, most private place I could find. I fell to the floor shaking and gasping uncontrollably. Tears welled up and overflowed. My hands and feet were ice cold. The shakes lasted for several minutes.

Afterwards, I felt oddly calm and relaxed. My mind was quiet and at peace. My body was free of tension, and I was able to sit cross-legged and comfortably fold my torso completely over my legs in repose. I later learned that I had experienced a Somatic Emotional Response to the change in my habitual breathing patterns. Emotional trauma from my past had been stored in the deep tissues of my body. The release of muscular tension brought about by changes in my breathing pattern caused the release of long stored emotion.

Although this emotion was not attached to a specific memory and occurred out of context with the events that created it, the experience of the emotional expression and release was profoundly physical. From that moment I began a personal exploration of exactly how my breathing was serving me in my life. Now that I knew what could happen as a result of exploring breath change, I could invite the release and open myself to what it could teach me about myself. While I had been intellectually aware that my breath was diminished and often shallow (I had a habit of sighing often to get more oxygen) I was not aware of the profound emotional implications of my breathing pattern. The ability to connect my breathing with my self-expression was a dramatic life change. I understand now that by diminishing my breath, I was literally limiting how much of the outer world I took in. The pattern began as a protective mechanism and eventually became unconscious and habitual. The experience of physical, emotional and mental change that occurred as a result of a change in my breathing led to a change in the relationship between my inner world and the outer world.

While a change in a part changes the Whole, the context in which a pattern occurs is also important to the **WholeMovement** Approach. Consider the story of "Back Man".

Back Man

Chronic back pain is a very common problem in today's modern world. When in pain a person may try to mask the pain with medication, or avoid it by not moving. In extreme cases the person may resort to surgery. As practitioners of **WholeMovement**, we frequently see individuals who have tried the obvious "fixes" without results and are seeking to avoid the extreme of a surgical procedure.

Back Man had tried pain pills, chiropractors, physical therapists, acupuncture and massage. Each intervention may have provided some short-term relief, but the pattern of pain kept returning. When Back Man agreed to try **WholeMovement**, he felt he had nothing to lose. In observing the characteristics of Back Man's personal movement signature, it was evident that he was an experienced and capable mover in good over-all physical condition. His movement expression was dominantly Bound Flow, with a Sudden use of Time. In binding his Flow he was expressing his reliance on internal muscular control. Sudden Time supported him by providing momentum for propelling the body. In other words, he was more focused on the *what* and *how* components of movement, rather than the *where*. The mechanics of body action were in the foreground of his movement signature, while his use and awareness of Space was diminished.

In a **WholeMovement** experience, Back Man was given the opportunity to more fully experience the spatial aspects of his movement. As a result he was able to increase his access to the full range of his flow, with less over-reliance on Bound Flow. Bringing him to an awareness of his environment allowed him to experience a balance of exertion and recuperation. It also allowed him to experience the connection between the workings of his inner world and the surrounding environment. His tendency to over stabilize through muscular control and momentum was moderated, thus breaking the cycle of chronic back pain. Now, rather than looking for a fix of the symptom of back pain, he sees the bigger picture and is able to recognize and adjust patterns of movement that cause the onset of pain. This is a good example of how back pain cannot be addressed as a problem in isolation; it must be considered within the context of the whole pattern in which it occurs.

In **WholeMovement** we recognize that the functionality and expressiveness of movement are intertwined. It is possible to change a movement pattern from either perspective. The Function/Expression connection is well illustrated in "Powerless Girl's" story.

Powerless Girl

When Powerless Girl was enrolled in a modern dance class she was unable to perform movements that required her to use her hands against the floor to push her body. One particular movement involved rolling the body from lying on the belly to sitting. The way to optimize this movement is to push from the upper body to propel the rotation to sitting. Powerless Girl rolled and then sat, without pushing. This inhibited her ability to do the movement smoothly and quickly. While she was able to perform the action successfully when individually coached by the teacher, when she was left on her own, she returned to her old preferential pattern. Her movement signature clearly demonstrated that she was not comfortable with any action that she perceived as pushy. When following orders, it was okay to be pushy, but when she was in charge, she opted out. In this case, what was needed was for her to be able to understand the necessity to focus on the functional aspect of movement rather than the personal aspect of what it expressed for her. Sometimes we are unaware of how our movement patterns reflect our attitudes and cultural beliefs, many times inhibiting our full functionality and expressive potential.

The connection between Function/Expression can be illustrated from another perspective. Achieving a functional goal can be enhanced when one acknowledges the expressive intention behind it. In **WholeMovement** we understand that clarifying the intention of movement will clarify the result. Not all **WholeMovement** interventions are concerned with chronic pain. Sometimes it is about optimizing and enhancing physical performance, as well as personal growth and development. The story of "Power Girl" illustrates this.

Power Girl

"Power Girl" was a performing artist, both a dancer and actor. She was enrolled in a class based on experiential anatomy. The class was working on weight shift and was doing an exercise that challenged her to move her pelvis directly forward from a sitting position to a kneeling position. She was having difficulty with this move and was focused on the functional action of the hip joint. She was frustrated because, as a competent mover, she didn't understand why she couldn't accomplish this weight shift when the students around her were moving with apparent ease. Her frustration triggered a defiant response, resulting in her accomplishing the forward pelvic shift. She froze for a moment with a look of total surprise on her face and blurted out, "it feels so aggressive!" Her own personal sense of the expressiveness of this movement allowed her to repeat it. No amount of focus on the functional aspect of the hip joint was going to work for her until she could be aware of movement's expressive capacity and the personal meaning it had for her.

WholeMovement is a way to repattern movement. It is not about replacing one pattern with another, it is about recognizing our personal preferences and understanding when and how they either serve or inhibit us. *WholeMovement* opens the door to alternatives, expanding and optimizing our potential as functional and expressive human beings. "Karen's Story" illustrates an aspect of her personal preference in phrasing style.

Karen's Story

While I was participating in a class on movement phrasing, we were directed in a task to stack and unstack chairs in order to observe each other's phrasing style. One member of the group was to stack and unstack folding chairs for a designated time period while the other members of the group observed. I was first. When the clock started ticking, I began stacking and unstacking the chairs as quickly as I could, and accelerated throughout the duration of the process. By the end, I was exhausted and relieved that my turn was over! Unconsciously I had approached the task from a "more is better/race against time" perspective.

The next member of my group approached the task in a very different way. Not at all in a hurry, she strolled among the chairs and then proceeded to playfully and artfully experiment with how they might be stacked and unstacked: upside down, one on top of the other, facing one way, facing another. My response was one of horror at myself! Why had I not thought that there was another way to do this? This experience illustrated a much bigger pattern of imbalance in Exertion/Recuperation in my life. My performance during this task clearly mirrored my tendency to drive myself to the point of exhaustion and collapse, never allowing myself to recuperate. Recuperation for me was a necessity brought on by exhaustion, rather than a choice. This phrasing pattern diminished the quality of my life. Finding the inherent pleasure in a more balanced approach to exertion and recuperation led to more conscious choices in how I approach tasks. It is not always about more and faster equals better.

Experiencing yourself through movement, and recognizing your personal movement patterns can lead to personal growth and development. This may include freeing yourself from chronic pain, deepening your awareness of your personal beliefs and value systems, and feeling more comfortable in your own skin as a physical body who moves.

EveryBody has a Story

APPENDIX A

Overview of Movement Analysis

The **WholeMovement** approach to movement education (training, re-patterning, intervention) evolved from the authors' work as practicing Certified Movement Analysts (CMA). One becomes a CMA through rigorous training in Laban Movement Analysis (LMA), a program of the Laban/Bartenieff Institute of Movement Studies.

Rudolf Laban (1879 - 1958) is best known for his system of dance notation (Labanotation). Labanotation is analogous to music notation, and is primarily used for recording and reconstructing dances in the same way that music notation is used to record and reconstruct musical compositions. Labanotation, however, is just a tiny fraction of Laban's work, which included the arts, education, industry and multiple other aspects of the study of human movement. Laban was a multi-dimensional thinker, practitioner, theorist and philosopher whose work influenced choreography, anthropology, psychology and other fields of human movement, and continues to reverberate and expand today.

One of his best-known students and protégés was Irmgard Bartenieff (1900 -1981). She was an educator, physical therapist and also a pioneer in the field of Dance Therapy. Bartenieff's own development of Laban's work, called Bartenieff Fundamentals™ (BF), resulted in the creation of what is now known as The Laban/Bartenieff Institute of Movement Studies, and the development of the Certification Program in Laban Movement Analysis. Bartenieff's work is a further application and delineation of Laban's work; one can understand LMA through Bartenieff Fundamentals™ and vice versa, leading to the authors' case for changing the current, separate LMA and BF acronyms to LBMS (Laban/Bartenieff Movement System).

Laban/Bartenieff Movement System (LBMS) is a comprehensive system used in understanding multiple aspects of human movement patterns. Its methodology incorporates a theoretical framework and clearly delineated language for movement. This language consists of a comprehensive, codified vocabulary. The LBMS is used to identify, record and interpret both macro and micro patterns of human movement. As a system of movement analysis, LBMS is unique, as it identifies and codifies both the qualitative as well as quantitative aspects of movement. In other words, the system takes into account both the functional as well as expressive content of actions. The system is also capable of identifying and differentiating what are universal patterns common to all humans; to group patterns (including cultural); and patterns that identify unique characteristics of an individual. The LBMS continues to develop and evolve hand in hand with current research and development across disciplines.

All systems of analysis are based on the identification of patterns. LBMS addresses patterns of movement in three distinct ways. One is the overall interplay within Themes of Duality. These movement dualities are identified as: Function/Expression, Stability/Mobility, Exertion/Recuperation and Inner/Outer. Other thematic dualities are also part of LBMS. Examples of these include Self/Other, Macro/Micro, Simple/Complex, Change/Constant. The list of thematic dualities is actually limitless, because all of these themes can be linked to the overarching duality of Part/Whole.

The second pattern LBMS addresses is the Phrasing of movement. Phrases are discreet, identifiable patterns of movement that are essential parts of larger patterns of movement. Phrases are specific units of movement which progress from a beginning to an ending. Phrasing organizes movement into recognizable forms.

The third characteristic pattern is the Developmental Progression of movement. These patterns can be recognized from many different perspectives, from the basic progression of individual motor development, to the larger perspective of human development over time.

Each of the three large patterns of movement described above is a big construct under which smaller components of movement can be grouped. Human movement is a multi-layered phenomenon, including relational aspects of the mover to themselves and to their environment supported by body organization and the nuance of subtle shifts in dynamics. This is why many versions of "body language" are so incapable of describing the precision and subtlety of our primary mode of communication and expression. LBMS recognizes the combinations of variables which account for why the same gesture or same action can be interpreted in one case as, powerful and assertive, while in another, as timid or lacking authenticity.

The Laban/Bartenieff Movement Analysis System breaks down human movement into four primary components: **Body, Effort, Shape** and **Space**. These components are linked to the what, where, how and why of action. Each of these components can be individually identified but all are also understood to be contextually interwoven, and that the relational aspects of these components is critical to understanding the meaningfulness of movement patterns. The appendices that follow are intended for students of LBMS, and incorporate specific terms (words that appear in capitals) and symbols used in this system.

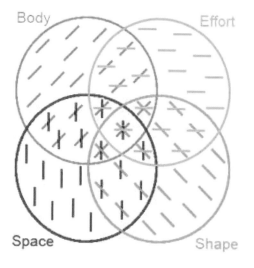

Model by Karen Studd

APPENDIX B

Motif - Capturing the Essence Symbolically

In addition to the comprehensive language, LBMS also utilizes a visual symbolic representation of movement. This pictorial representation is called Motif Writing, and was originally derived from Labanotation. Motif symbols are used to capture the most salient aspects of a movement event, in contrast to Labanotation, which is used to record all the details of an event.

The purpose of Motif Writing is to capture the essence of movement, conveying overall meaning. In the LBMS system Motif Writing can be used in a number of ways, including:

- A quick shorthand when words prove too cumbersome

- A catalyst in the observation process, requiring the observer to choose what is most important about a movement event, thus revealing larger patterns.

- A vehicle to free a mover from habitual or preferential patterns

- A method for reaching observer consensus about a movement event establishing validity

- To reveal what is missing

- To clarify what is most essential in a movement event

Motive writing occurs in two forms: vertical and horizontal. In the horizontal orientation the symbols reveal the sequence in which a series of actions occurs, and only allows the representation of one action at a time. The vertical orientation allows for more complexity, including duration of actions and simultaneous actions.

Motif begins with a symbol called the Action stroke, a simple vertical line upon which all other symbols are derived. The Action stroke shows the difference between action and no-action, and its length is an indication of relative time. Empty space between action strokes means no action is occurring. In the vertical motif example below, four actions occur. The first action is followed by a pause and takes twice as long to occur as the three actions that follow it.

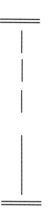

In the preceding example, there is no indication of the type of movement change occurring. To further augment and clarify a movement event, action strokes may be replaced by more specific symbols in each of the categories of Body, Effort, Space and Shape.

The general symbol representing Body   8

The general symbol representing Effort   /

The general symbol representing Space   []

The general symbol for Shape   //

In each of these categories the general symbol can be made more specific and combined with other symbols.

In the Appendices which follow, we have included samples of commonly used Motif symbols.

APPENDIX C

The Body Component of LBMS

In LBMS, the "what" of movement is the **Body** component. Body describes how the body is organized, specific body parts and actions, and what is emphasized. This component also reveals aspects of movement motivation and intent. Categories include:

Basic anatomy/physiology as it relates to movement
Body Parts
Patterns of Body Organization
Basic Body Actions
Bartenieff Fundamentals™
Body Connections
Body Rhythms

Motif Man – Body Parts

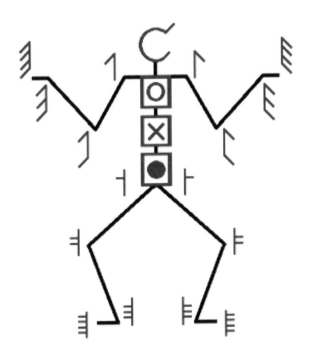

Appendix C

Patterns of Body Organization

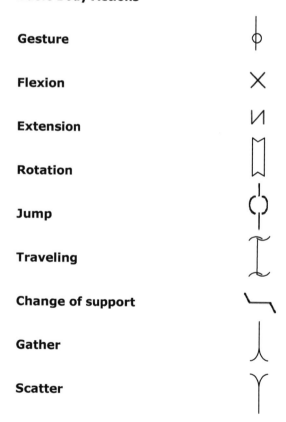

Core-Distal

Head-Tail

Upper-Lower

Right-Left

Cross-Lateral

The patterns and symbols above can also be found in "Making Connections: Total Body Integration Through Bartenieff Fundamentals" by Peggy Hackney

Basic Body Actions

Gesture

Flexion

Extension

Rotation

Jump

Traveling

Change of support

Gather

Scatter

In the above list each of these basic symbols can be further delineated. For example, the symbol for rotation can be made more specific, becoming the symbol for a turn or a twist.

Bartenieff Fundamentals™ (BF)

Bartenieff Fundamentals™ address optimizing the supportive relationship between body organization and movement intention. It incorporates Fundamental Principles and specific movement sequences, such as The Basic Six Exercises (see below). BF is supported by the theory and embodiment of Laban Space Harmony. It is a tool that can be used for movement re-patterning (originally Irmgard Bartenieff's "Correctives"), to expand, enhance and maintain movement capacity throughout one's life.

BF Principles

The following list is not necessarily hierarchical (although it is common to experience breath as the starting point) because each one of the Principles is inherently related to all the rest (Part/Whole).

- **Breath Support** – The quality, rhythm, duration and volume of breath supports all aspects of movement. The anatomical/physiological design of the breathing process is core to the experience of being human. Comprehension of this Principle also includes the nature of the breath process as both being conscious and volitional, as well as unconscious and automatic. Breath is the Basis of the Inner/Outer LBMS Theme.

- **Axis of Length** – a primary given of our human design, it defines our bilateral symmetry. Throughness of the axis of length is necessary for Whole body connectivity. (NB The authors' have added this Principle to their list of BF Principles)

- **Dynamic Alignment** – seeks to optimize the functional efficiency of the ongoing changing relationships of body parts as we move. This principle focuses on skeletal connections to optimize the patterning of kinetic chains.

- **Core Support** – The core of the body is the essence of self and core support is about uniting all deep aspects of self. This recognizes that core anatomy is linked to self-identity, including such things as core beliefs and intentions. Bringing a deep muscular-skeletal-organ involvement to our movement enables us to commit our entire selves to movement.

- **Developmental Pattern Support** – The patterned progression of limb/core relationships as the underpinning of all human movement. Developmental stages as building blocks in fundamental body organization.

- **Weight Shift from the Pelvic Core** – to support the human design for locomotion.

- **Body Level Phrasing** – initiation (core, proximal, mid-limb, distal) and sequencing (Simultaneous, Sequential, Successive) of action in support of movement intent.

- **Rotary Support** – joint rotation as a fundamental component of complex three-dimensional movement; necessary for adaptation, accommodation and interaction.

- **Spatial Intent** – clarifying the Functional and Expressive relationship between Body organization and spatial goals.

- **Effort Intent** – clarifying the relationship between motivation and action, and optimizing the mover's intention through awareness of dynamic choices.

- **Shape Intent** – support for action in the mover's change of form relative to self and the environment.

The Basic 6

The Basic 6 are movement sequences that allow the mover to focus on fundamental body connections. These are not set "exercises", but rather patterns to be used as an inroad to exploring and refining movement. These sequences can also be used diagnostically to identify the mover's preferential patterns and restrictions.

- Thigh lift – (ilio-femoral rhythm) the flexion and extension of the hip joint, which connects the lower limb to the core. This pattern supports locomotion and level change.

- Sagittal Pelvic Shift – mobilization of the pelvis through a core to limb connection for efficient forward locomotion and centering weight over the base of support.

- Lateral Pelvic Shift – mobilization of the pelvis through a core to limb connection for efficient lateral weight shift and support.

- Body Half – connecting the upper and lower body through the process of differentiating the right and left sides of the body as established through the spinal midline.

- Contralateral Knee Drop (aka, Knee Reach) – basis of the contralateral rotary connection between the upper and lower body.

- Arm Circle – (Scapulo-Humeral rhythm) maximizing the three-dimensional rotational capacity of the upper body, and connection of the upper limb to the core.

It should be noted that, in addition to the Basic Six listed above, there are other movement sequences associated with Bartenieff Fundamentals, such as Heel Rock and X-rolls. There are many ways of exploring the Basic Six and associated movement sequences.

APPENDIX D

The Effort Component of LBMS

The term "Effort" (a translation of the German "antrieb") tells us "how" a movement is performed. Effort describes the dynamic or qualitative aspects of the movement. Dynamics give the feel, texture, tone, or color of the movement and illuminate the mover's attitude, inner intent, and how they exert and organize their energy. Effort is in constant flux and modulation, with Factors combining together in different combinations of two or three, and shifting in intensity throughout the progression of movement. These combinations of Effort occur in sequences called phrases. The quality of phrases is determined by where emphasis occurs through loading or accenting. The Effort component includes:

Effort Factors (four)
Effort Elements (eight)
States (six)
Drives (four)
Phrasing Types:
- Even – no emphasis
- Impactive – emphasis at the end
- Impulsive – emphasis at the beginning
- Swing – emphasis in the middle

Effort Factors – each with two contrasting Elements

Effort Factors	Indulging Element	Condensing Element
Flow *Progression/Feeling*	**Free** *released ongoingness*	**Bound** *controlled ongoingness*
Weight *Intention/Sensing*	**Light** *delicate*	**Strong** *forceful*
Space *Attention/Thinking*	**Indirect** *expansive outer awareness*	**Direct** *channeled outer awareness*
Time *Commitment/Deciding*	**Sustained** *lingering*	**Quick** *urgent*

Effort Graph

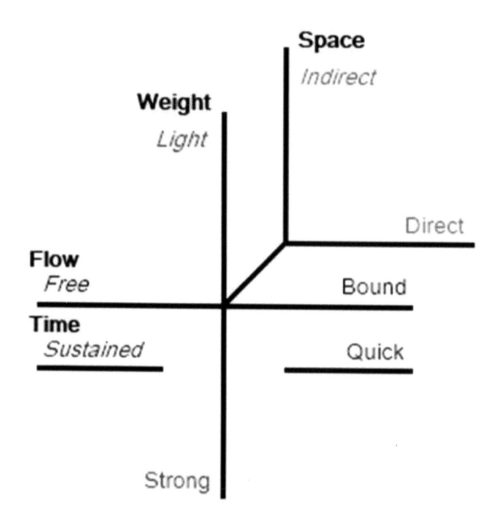

Combinations of two Effort Factors are called States. There are six States, each with four combinations of two Effort Elements. Combinations of three Effort Factors are called Drives. There are Four Drives, each with eight combinations of three Effort Elements.

The six States are:

Dream (Weight/Flow)　　　　　　**Awake** (Time/Space)

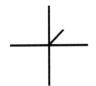　　　　　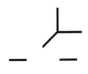

Rhythm, aka Near (Weight/Time)　　**Remote**, aka Far (Space/Flow)

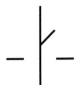　　　　　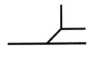

Mobile (Time/Flow)　　　　　　**Stable** (Weight/Space)

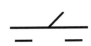　　　　　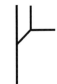

Note that the six States above are listed in pairs with opposing Effort Factors. Each State is expressed in four possible configurations. For example, Dream State can be: Strong/Bound, or Strong/Free, or Light/Bound, or Light/Free.

The four Drives are:

Action (Weight/Time/Space)   **Spell** (Flow/Weight/Space)

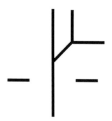   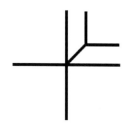

Vision (Flow/Time/Space)   **Passion** (Flow/Weight/Time)

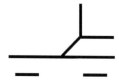   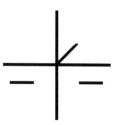

    Each Drive has one Factor missing. For example, Action Drive has no Flow. The missing Factor can be as significant as the three Factors that are present in the Expression of movement. Each Drive is expressed in eight possible configurations. In Action Drive these eight are named: Float, Punch, Glide, Slash, Flick, Press, Dab and Wring.

    There is harmony in the relationships of Effort. Each Factor has an oppositional pair of elements. The States can be paired as opposites. Each State is associated with a pair of Drives. For example, Stable State is a shared component of Action Drive and Spell Drive.

Effort Factors with States and Drives

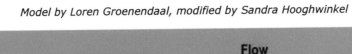

Model by Loren Groenendaal, modified by Sandra Hooghwinkel

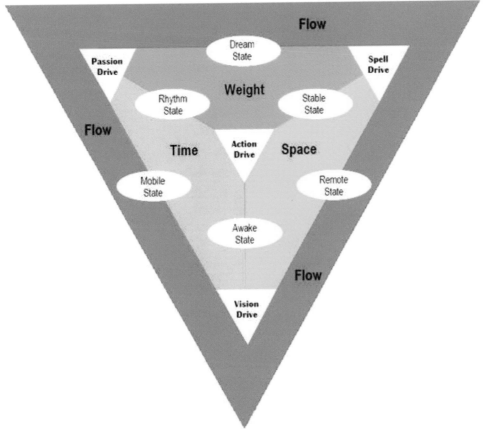

APPENDIX E

The Space Component of LBMS

Space references the overall environment, as well as the mover's personal space. Space looks at such distinctions as direction, level, pathways, tensions and counter tensions of actions. Space reveals the trajectories and inclinations of paths of action. Laban's theories of Space Harmony (Choreutics) include the practice of movement scales (similar to scales in music) within the architecture of crystalline shapes, including the octahedron, the icosahedron and the cube. The Space Component includes:

Directions – 26 directions from Place Middle
- 6 Dimensional Directions
- 12 Planal Directions
- 8 Diagonal Directions

Kinesphere Reach Space
- Near-reach
- Mid-reach
- Far-reach

Polyhedral Forms
- Tetrahedron
- Octahedron
- Cube
- Icosahedron
- Dodecahedron

Scales of the Polyhedra
- Dimensional and Defense (Octahedron)
- Diagonal (Cube)
- Axis, Girdle, Primary, A and B (Icosahedron)

Approach to Kinesphere and Pathways
- Central
- Peripheral
- Transverse

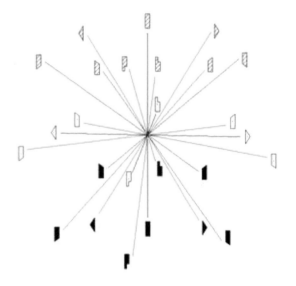

26 directions from Place Middle, Model by Sandra Hooghwinkel

Polyhedra – Models of Platonic Solids

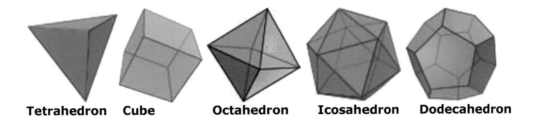

Tetrahedron   **Cube**   **Octahedron**   **Icosahedron**   **Dodecahedron**

Directional Symbols

		Left/Forward/High	Forward/High	Right/Forward/High
High Level		Left/High	Place High	Right/High
		Left/Back/High	Back/High	Right/Back/High
		Left/Forward/Middle	Forward/Middle	Right/Forward/Middle
Middle Level		Left/Middle	Place Middle	Right/Middle
		Left/Back/Middle	Back/Middle	Right/Back/Middle
		Left/Forward/Low	Forward/Low	Right/Forward/Low
Low Level		Left/Low	Place Low	Right/Low
		Left/Back/Low	Back/Low	Right/Back/Low

Cross of Axes with Symbols

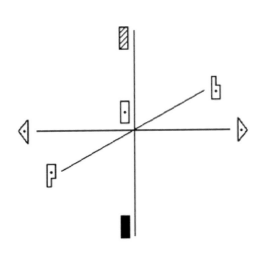

Planes

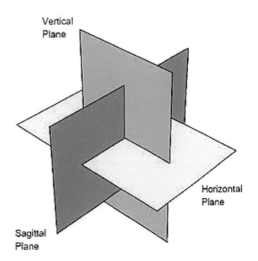

Cube with Diagonal Symbols

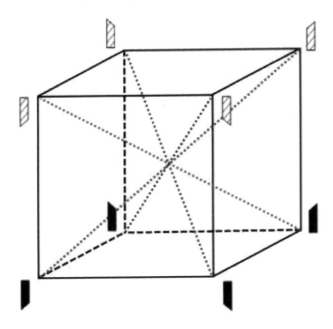

APPENDIX F

The Shape Component of LBMS

Shape addresses how the changing form of the mover relates to themselves and/or to their environment. The Shape Flow of movement can be seen in the adjustments and actions of attending to oneself – shifting weight, repositioning, and actions of self-reference. The mover also uses the form of their shape to bridge to their environment as they reach, point, or push. Movers may also accommodate their form to something or someone else, drawing on the ability to mold and adapt their form in a mutual relationship. Shape indicates aspects of object relationship and the locus of control. Qualities of the mover's changing Shape also convey information about the ongoing connection between the mover's inner and outer worlds.

Shape Component includes:

Still Shape Forms (sometimes referred to simply as Shape Forms)

- Wall

- Ball

- Pin

- Screw

- Tetrahedron

Modes of Shape Change

- Shape Flow

- Directional Movement
  - Spoke-like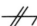

  - Arc-like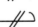

- Shaping (Carving)

Appendix F

Shape Qualities

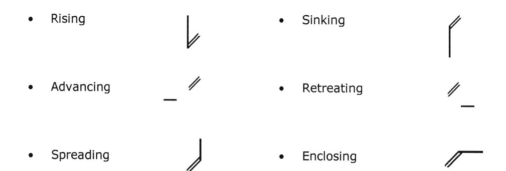

- Rising

- Sinking

- Advancing

- Retreating

- Spreading

- Enclosing

Shape Qualities Graph

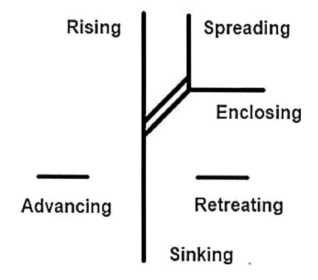

148

APPENDIX G

Synthesis: Returning the Parts To the Whole

Analysis and synthesis are another Part/Whole duality that is related to the meaningfulness of movement. While human movement can be broken down into parts through analysis, it can only be understood in returning the parts to the Whole through the process of synthesis. Micro patterns of the components of movement (Body, Effort, Space, Shape) reveal the meaningfulness of movement when brought into relationship with the Macro patterns of Thematic Dualities, Phrasing and Developmental Progression. In LBMS the concept of Space Harmony addresses the synthesis of the Part/Whole relationship.

Space Harmony

LBMS includes the study and practice of ordered movement sequences through space called Scales. These spatial scales are analogous to musical scales of tonal progression. The scales occur within the larger architecture of space, which can be identified through the models of the Platonic Solids. The scales are used to illuminate the space harmony of movement, connecting the changing form of the body in its dynamic expression through space. The Dimensional Cross of Axes and the Defense Scale occur within the Octahedron. The Diagonal Scale occurs within the Cube. The Axis, Girdle, Primary, A and B scales are examples of Icosahedral Scales. Spatial relationships can be identified between and among each of the scales. For instance, an Axis Scale of the Icosahedron is linked to one of the Diagonals of the Cube. In addition, the Platonic Solids themselves exist in dual relationships to one another.

There are patterns that can be identified through the harmonic relationships among Body, Effort, Shape and Space. For example, the six Dimensional Directions are correlated with what are termed Affinities. This relationship is outlined in the table below.

Shape Quality	Effort Element	Spatial Aspect
Rising	Light Weight	High
Sinking	Strong Weight	Low
Advancing	Sustained Time	Forward
Retreating	Quick Time	Backward
Spreading	Indirect	Side Open
Enclosing	Direct	Side Across

The harmonic relationships listed above arise from the experience of the moving body. For example, Light Weight Effort while Rising upward is directly linked to the experience of the Center of Levity, located in the upper body. Sinking downward with Strong Weight is correlated with the Center of Gravity, located in the lower body. Our dominant mode of perception for attending to the environment is our vision. Access to peripheral vision supports the expression of Indirect Space Effort, while foveal vision supports the expression of Direct Space Effort. The body is the basis for each one of the above relationships.

Just as dissonance is a powerful expression in music, disaffined movement of the body's dynamics in space is also powerful and can be considered the dual expression of the affined patterns. Space Harmony speaks to the balance and Wholeness of human movement.

The Dynamosphere

Expression does not occur in a vacuum. It occurs in the environment through which we move. The Dynamosphere is a more macro concept than the Kinesphere in that it links Effort with Space. It is a container for the energies of all human movement and goes beyond the boundaries of the individual mover's Kinesphere into the shared general space. The Dynamosphere is another aspect of Space Harmony, connecting the parts of movement expression to the Whole of movement expression.

Development and Applications of Rudolf Laban's work

Like any moving system, LBMS continues to grow and develop. Many individuals have made significant contributions to the ongoing progression of the work of Rudolf Laban. The list of possible applications of this work are varied, far-reaching and occur in every domain of human movement (which is to say, everywhere in everything!). Some examples include:

- Therapeutic Interventions (Psychotherapy, Dance Therapy, Occupational Therapy, etc.)

- Conflict Resolution

- The human movement interface with science and technology

- Coaching and training (athletes, dancers, actors, musicians, public speakers)

- Education – the movement aspect of learning and knowing

- Somatics, health and well-being practices

- Arts and Architecture

- Cultural anthropology

- Comparative analysis

- Skills training and functional efficiency

- Animation and Motion Capturing

Authors' Bios

Karen A. Studd, holds a Master of Science degree from University of Oregon. In addition Karen is a CMA (Certified Movement Analyst) and RSMT (Registered Somatic Movement Therapist and Registered Somatic Movement Educator (RSME). For twenty years she has taught and coordinated programs in Movement Analysis through the Laban/Bartenieff Institute for Movement Studies across the United States, Canada and Europe. In addition, she has taught workshops and presented papers in Poland, Brazil, and Slovakia.

Karen has been a faculty member of the University of Wisconsin, George Washington University and George Mason University, where she is a tenured faculty of the School of Dance and an affiliated faculty member for the Center for Consciousness and Transformation. A teacher of movement studies, experiential anatomy, dance technique, and a choreographer, she is focused on adult education and personal development through movement. Her interest is in promoting awareness of the body of knowledge of human movement across all disciplines. For the last several years Karen has been interested in movement as a component of leadership and has been sought out as a "body language expert" in the observation of the movement profiles of political pundits. She has been interviewed by the Washington Post newspaper, National Public Radio's "With Good Reason" and appeared on television's Hard Ball commentary with Chris Matthews.

Laura L. Cox, holds a Master of Arts degree in Dance and Dance Education from New York University. In addition Laura is also a CMA (Certified Movement Analyst) and RSME (Registered Somatic Movement Educator) and RSMT (Registered Somatic Movement Therapist) through the International Somatic Movement Education and Therapy Association (ISMETA). Her work is influenced by her studies in the somatic disciplines of Ideokinesis, Continuum and Zero Balancing. Currently she has a private practice in movement education and specializes in re-patterning the movement of clients suffering from chronic pain or injury. Her clients span the range from professionals in dance, sports and fitness to those with little or no movement experience. She is a teacher of dance technique, kinesiology, and movement health and well-being and has served on the faculties for New York University, The University of Nebraska, Towson University and The University of Maryland. In addition to her private practice, she currently teaches for the Laban/Bartenieff Institute of Movement Studies and conducts workshops and seminars in movement awareness and health. Laura is also an avid equestrian and has assisted in Therapeutic Riding programs.

References and related sources

Allison, Nancy, Editor, *The Complete Body, Mind, and Spirit*, Keats Publishing, originally published by The Rosen Publishing Group, Inc., 1999.

Bartenieff, Irmgard, with Dori Lewis, *Body Movement: Coping with the Environment*, Gordon and Breach Science Publishers, New York, 1980.

Bloomer, Kent C., Charles W. Moore and Robert J. Yudell, *Body, Memory and Architecture*, Yale University, 1977.

Bradley, Karen K., *Rudolf Laban*, Routledge Performance Practitioners, 2009.

Burton, John W., *Culture and the Human Body*, Waveland Press, Inc., 2001.

Calais-Germain, Blandine, *Anatomy of Movement*, Eastland Press, Inc., Seattle, Washington, 1993.

Cohen, Bonnie Bainbridge, *Sensing, Feeling and Action: The Experiential Anatomy of Body-Mind Centering*, Contact Editions, Northampton, Mass., 1993.

Damasio, Antonio R., *Descartes' Error: Emotion, Reason, and the Human Brain*, A Grosset/Putnam Book, NY, 1994.

Dowd, Irene, *Taking Root to Fly: Articles on Functional Anatomy*, Irene Dowd, New York, NY., 1996.

Hackney, Peggy, *Making Connections: Total Body Integration Through Bartenieff Fundamentals*, Gordon and Breach Publishers, 1998.

Hartley, Linda, *Wisdom of the Body Moving: An Introduction to Body-Mind Centering*, North Atlantic Books, Berkeley, CA, 1995.

Laban, Rudolf, *A Vision of Dynamic Space*, The Falmer Press, Philadelphia, PA, 1984.

Laban, Rudolf, *Choreutics*, MacDonald and Evans, London, 1966; 1st American ed., *The Language of Movement: A Guidebook to Choreutics*. Annotated and edited by Lisa Ullmann, Boston: Plays, Inc., 1974, c 1966.

Laban, Rudolf, *The Mastery of Movement*, MacDonald and Evans Limited, 1975 edition.

Lakoff, George and Mark Johnson, *Metaphors We Live By*, The University of Chicago Press, Chicago, 1980.

Lakoff, George and Mark Johnson, *Philosophy in the Flesh: The Embodied Mind and It's Challenge to Western Thought*, Basic Books, a member of the Perseus Books Group, 1999.

References and Related Sources

Lawlor, Robert, *Sacred Geometry: Philosophy and Practice*, Thames and Hudson Ltd., London, 1982.

Lehrer, Jonah, *Proust was a Neuroscientist*, First Mariner Books ed., 2008.

Moore, Carol-Lynne and Kaoru Yamamoto, *Beyond Words: Movement Observation and Analysis*, Gordon and Breach Science Publishers S.A., 1988.

Olsen, Andrea and Caryn McHose, *Body Stories: A Guide to Experiential Anatomy*, Station Hill Press, Barrytown, NY, 1991.

Preston-Dunlop, Valerie, *Rudolf Laban: An Extraordinary Life*, Dance Books Ltd., London, Great Britain, 1998.

Shlain, Leonard, *Art and Physics: Parallel Visions in Space, Time and Light*, Harper Collins Publishers Inc. 2001, Leonard Shlain, 1991.

Shlain, Leonard, *The Alphabet Versus the Goddess*, Arkana, Penguin Putnam Inc., 1999

Skinner, Stephen, *Sacred Geometry: Deciphering the Code*, Sterling Publishing Co., Inc., 2006.

Wilbur, Ken, *No Boundary: Eastern and Western Approaches to Personal Growth*, Shambhala Publications, Inc., Boston, Mass., 1979, 2001.

Williams, Terry Tempest, *Finding Beauty in a Broken World,* Pantheon, Random House, New York, 2008

Image references and sources

Atomic Particles
> Source/Author: From www.wpclipart.com [Public domain]

Planets Orbiting
> Source/Author: From www.suite101.com [Public domain]

Flowing River
> Source/Author: By Vincent (Personal picture) [Public domain], via Wikimedia Commons

Vehicular flow of traffic
> Source/Author: By Tomás Rodríguez Ontiveros (Own work) [CC-BY-SA-2.5], via Wikimedia Commons

YingYang
> Source/Author: By Kenny Shen (Derivative work) [Public domain], via Wikimedia Commons

Tightrope walker
> Source/Author: By Rhett Sutphin [CC-BY-2.0], via Wikimedia Commons

Lateral view of the dome shape of the Diaphragm
> Source/Author: By Pearson Scott Foresman [Public domain], via Wikimedia Commons

Thoracic diaphragm seen from below, with crura attached to spine
> Source/Author: From the 20th U.S. edition of Gray's Anatomy of the Human Body by Henry Gray, originally published in 1918 [Public domain], via Wikimedia Commons

Interrelationship of Iliopsoas and Thoracic Diaphragm
> Source/Author: By Michaël Nisand (Own work) [Public domain], via Wikimedia Commons

Old fashioned balance scales
> Source/Author: By Deutsche Fotothek [CC-BY-SA-3.0-de], via Wikimedia Commons

Vertical upright posture
> Source/Author: By Robert Gaudenzi (1842-1889) (Royal Library, Copenhagen) [Public domain], via Wikimedia Commons

Off vertical posture
> Source/Author: By Américo Nunes from Recife, Brasil (Nascer do Sol em Porto de Galinhas) [CC-BY-SA-2.0], via Wikimedia Commons

Moving skeletons
> Source/Author: From www.ClipartPal.com [Public domain]

Image References and Sources

Curves of spine
> Source/Author: By Sue Clark (Flickr: pg 192 Skull and Spine) [Public domain], via Wikimedia Commons

Star fish
> Source/Author: From the U.S. National Oceanic and Atmospheric Administration [Public domain], via Wikimedia Commons

Star angel
> Source/Author: By Kerys [CC-BY-2.0], via Wikimedia Commons

Snake
> Source/Author: By Konrad Lackerbeck (Own work) [CC-BY-3.0], via Wikimedia Commons

Belly Dancer
> Source/Author: By Jack Versloot (originally posted to Flickr as Belly Dancing) [CC-BY-2.0], via Wikimedia Commons

Frog
> Source/Author: By Keven Law from Los Angeles, USA [CC-BY-SA-2.0], via Wikimedia Commons

Diver
> Source/Author: By Werner100359 (Own work) [CC-BY-3.0], via Wikimedia Commons

Gecko
> Source/Author: By W.A. Djatmiko (Wie146) (Own work) [CC-BY-SA-3.0], via Wikimedia Commons

Rock climber
> Source/Author: By Robert Lawton [CC-BY-SA-2.5], via Wikimedia Commons

Runner in Aqua Sphere
> Source/Author: By Aquaspheres (Own work) [CC-BY-3.0], via Wikimedia Commons

Nordic walker
> Source/Author: By Malcolm Jarvis (Own work) [CC-BY-SA-3.0], via Wikimedia Commons

Spinning dancers
> Source/Author: By Ken Mayer (originally posted to Flickr as Jan twirling Beth) [CC-BY-2.0], via Wikimedia Commons

Rotation in nature
> Source/Author: Justin1569 at en.wikipedia [CC-BY-SA-3.0], via Wikimedia Commons

Rotation in architecture
> Source/Author: By Väsk (Own work) [CC-BY-SA-3.0], via Wikimedia Commons

Body rotation
> Source/Author: By MatthiasKabel (Roman bronze reduction of Myron's Discobolos, 2nd century CE) [CC-BY-SA-3.0], via Wikimedia Commons

Kiwis
> Source/Author: By J.smith (Own work) [CC-BY-SA-3.0], via Wikimedia Commons

Pelvis in relationship to spine
> Source/Author: From www.wpclipart.com [Public domain]

Pelvis in relation to lower limbs
> Source/Author: From www.wpclipart.com [Public domain]

Waterfall
> Source/Author: By David Tarazona (Archivo personal) [CC-BY-SA-3.0-2.5-2.0-1.0], via Wikimedia Commons

Frozen waterfall
> Source/Author: By Frank K. [CC-BY-2.0], via Wikimedia Commons

Heavy boulder
> Source/Author: By Michael Graham [CC-BY-SA-2.0], via Wikimedia Commons

Dandelion seeds
> Source/Author: By Hmbascom (Own work) [CC-BY-3.0], via Wikimedia Commons

Lightning
> Source/Author: By Lyoha123 (Own work) [CC-BY-SA-3.0], via Wikimedia Commons

Sunset
> Source/Author: By MAURO Didier (Own work) [CC-BY-SA-3.0-2.5-2.0-1.0], via Wikimedia Commons

Pressure washer
> Source/Author: I, Mschel [CC-BY-SA-3.0], via Wikimedia Commons

Wave hitting rock
> Source/Author: By Pöllö (Own work) [CC-BY-3.0], via Wikimedia Commons

Mobius strip
> Source/Author: By David Benbennick (Own work) [CC-BY-SA-3.0], via Wikimedia Commons

Image References and Sources

Sculpture by Fernando Botero
> Source/Author: By Michael Mertens from Darmstadt, Germany (Goslar Rosentor Skulpturen) [CC-BY-SA-2.0], via Wikimedia Commons

Three Men Walking II, sculpture by Alberto Giacometti
> Source/Author: sculpture by Alberto Giacometti, 1949, Metropolitan Museum of Art, Bronze. [Fair Use Rationale], via Wikipedia.
> In this book on movement studies, the image is used to illustrate a specific example on the subject. Therefore we believe it constitutes fair use and does not infringe copyright.

Marilyn Monroe in spiral shape
> Source/Author: By Studio publicity still [Public domain], via Wikimedia Commons

Gestural Directional movement
> Source/Author: By User:Rodasmith (Photo by User:Rodasmith) [CC-BY-SA-3.0-2.5-2.0-1.0], via Wikimedia Commons

Postural Directional Movement
> Source/Author: By Sucheerraiders [CC-BY-SA-3.0], via Wikimedia Commons

Shaping clay
> Source/Author: By Soyer Isabelle at nl.wikipedia [CC-BY-2.0-be], via Wikimedia Commons

Runner breaking through the finish line
> Source/Author: By New York World-Telegram and the Sun Newspaper Photograph Collection. (NYPL Digital) [Public domain], via Wikimedia Commons

Adult embracing children
> Source/Author: By U.S. Navy photo by Mass Communication Specialist 1st Class Leah Stiles [Public domain], via Wikimedia Commons

Astronaut in space capsule
> Source/Author: By NASA [Public domain], via Wikimedia Commons

Astronaut performing spacewalk
> Source/Author: By NASA (Great Images in NASA Description) [Public domain], via Wikimedia Commons

Pointing forward
> Source/Author: By EricS at de.wikipedia (Original text : de:Benutzer:EricS) [CC-BY-SA-3.0], via Wikimedia Commons

Pointing sideways
> Source/Author: By golanlevin [CC-BY-2.0], via Wikimedia Commons

Child pushing grandmother
> Source/Author: By Catherine Scott (Matti) [CC-BY-SA-2.0], via Wikimedia Commons

Grandmother and grandchild playing with crayon
> Source/Author: By Roy Klomp (Own work)) [CC-BY-3.0]

INDEX

CPSIA information can be obtained
at www.ICGtesting.com
Printed in the USA
BVIC00n0640211213
339760BV00002B/2